Rosemary Stanton's

FAT & FIBRE COUNTER

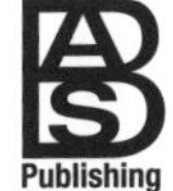

Published by:

BAS Publishing
ABN 30 106 181 542
PO Box 2052
Seaford Vic 3198
Tel/Fax: (03) 5988 3597

Web: www.baspublishing.com.au
Email: mail@baspublishing.com.au

The National Library of Australia Cataloguing-in-Publication entry

Stanton, Rosemary.
Rosemary Stanton's fat & fibre counter.

New ed.
ISBN 1 920910 26 3.

1. Food - Fat content - Tables. 2. Food - Fiber content - Tables. 3. Food - Calorie content - Tables. 4. Glycemic index. I. Title.

613.23

Page Layout: exigene.com.au
Cover Design: Selina Low

The Fat & Fibre Counter

The ideal diet is high in fibre and low in saturated fat, refined sugars and refined starches. Carbohydrates with a low Glycaemic Index (GI) are preferred, although the GI should not be used as the sole basis for judging a food.

You don't need to have everything bursting with fibre. Nor should you avoid all fat. You just need some balance – choosing the best fats and the best carbohydrates where possible. This book shows you how.

By eating less fat, more fibre and better quality carbohydrates, you can help normalise blood cholesterol and triglyceride levels, reduce excess body fat and also decrease your risk of coronary heart disease, bowel cancer, breast cancer, gall stones, diabetes and high blood pressure.

How To Use This Book

Fat

If you are overweight, follow the **30-40 guide** – aim for **30-40 grams of fat** and **30-40 grams of fibre** a day. Not all fats are equal and we've given you a quick guide with ticks and crosses. As you would expect, two ticks are better than one and two crosses are worse than one.

An occasional splurge doesn't hurt but even if you are not overweight, you should still avoid large quantities of saturated fat most of the time and try to keep your total day's fat intake to:

- 30-50 grams – for most women and children;
- 40-60 grams – for most men;
- 70 grams – for active teenagers and adults who are very active;
- 80-100 grams – if you do lots of physical activity at work (for example, bricklaying) or extensive athletic training (for example, triathlons or marathons).

(These figures are calculated to provide approximately 25% of kilojoules from fat – a level which is safe and adequate.)

Good fats/bad fats

✓ The food has 'good' (unsaturated) fats.

✓✓ The food has 'good' fat plus omega 3 fatty acids or makes a good contribution to other important nutrients.

✗✗ The food has 'bad' saturated fats present as more than a third of the fat.

✗ The total quantity of 'bad' fat is small or the food contributes worthwhile quantities of one or more other nutrients.

For example, a food such as cheese contains 'bad' saturated fats, but is valuable for its high content of calcium, protein and riboflavin, so it scores only one cross, whereas potato crisps have few valuable nutrients with their saturated fat and score two crosses. No crosses or ticks mean that the food contains very little fat (for example, vegetables or the milk in a cup of tea).

Kilojoules

Kilojoules do count, but counting them is rather tedious. A soundly-based weight loss eating pattern should have about 5000-6500 kJ. Eating less than this simply reduces the body's metabolic rate and makes you feel lethargic. If you prefer the older term kilocalories (usually written as Calories), 1Cal = 4.2kJ. To translate back from kilojoules to Calories, divide the figures given in this book by 4.2. For example, a slice of bread has 290 kJ, or 70 Cals.

Good carbs/bad carbs

✓ The food contains carbohydrates plus other important nutrients.

✓✓ Other important nutrients are present and the food has a low Glycaemic Index (GI).

✗ The food contains more than 1 teaspoon sugar or an equivalent amount of highly refined carbohydrate per serve.

✗✗ The food has a higher content of sugar or refined carbohydrate and no worthwhile quantities of any other nutrients.

Some points about GI

- GI refers to the rate at which the carbohydrate in the food is converted to blood glucose compared with straight glucose. Carbohydrates that are converted to glucose more slowly create less stress on blood sugar and insulin levels.
- GI refers only to foods that contain a certain amount of carbohydrate – usually 10g per serve. Foods such as many vegetables, herbs and salads vegetables do not have a GI because they have too little carbohydrate.

GI numbers are only accurate to plus or minus 9 Points and represent the average values obtained from approximately 10 healthy university students. I have therefore not included GI numbers but have given an extra tick to foods that fit into the category of low GI, as long as they also make a worthwhile nutritional contribution.

GI is also affected by the presence of fats, protein and certain types of fibre because these components delay the rate at which food is emptied from the stomach into the small intestine where the breakdown to glucose occurs.

Other factors that influence the GI include how much foods are chewed, different cooking techniques, the physical form of the food (for example whether it is stewed apple pieces or pureed apple), the integrity of the food (for example, if wheat grains are ground into stoneground wholemeal flour or whether the wholemeal flour has been recombined from white flour with added bran and wheatgerm) and the presence of acid ingredients (adding lemon juice or vinegar to a food reduces its GI).

GI should only be used to rate foods within a food group. For example, it is valid to choose a sour dough or wholegrain bread in preference to a white or wholemeal loaf, but it is not nutritionally valid to choose ice cream over carrots, just because ice cream has a lower GI.

In this guide, foods have been given two ticks in the Carb column only if they have a low GI and other important nutrients.

Fibre

For good health, everyone except babies, infants and small children should have about 30 to 40 grams of dietary fibre a day. For young children, an appropriate fibre intake is 5-10g plus their age.

Arrangement

All foods are arranged alphabetically. Where possible, realistic, average-sized serves have been used. Where values have been calculated from a recipe used by a restaurant or from a recipe book, they are on the basis of the stated number of servings for the recipe. If you eat unusually large or small portions, you will need to make appropriate adjustments.

All home-made items are from standard recipes. If you are dedicated to healthy cooking, you can make many dishes with less fat or less saturated fat. For example, if you make junket or custard with skim milk rather than regular milk, you will decrease the fat and kilojoules. If you use olive oil rather than butter or margarine for cooking, you won't decrease the amount of fat, but you will be choosing a better fat (a ✓ rather than a ✗). Fat content can also be reduced by using non-stick pans rather than adding oil or fat.

All figures have been rounded off. For fibre and fat, figures have been taken to the nearest half gram. For kilojoules, values have been rounded to the nearest 5. Where a cooked weight is given, it refers to the portion that will be eaten. For raw products, the weight is as purchased but the percentage of skin, pips or other inedible parts has been taken into account. For example, a passionfruit weighing 40g has 20g of edible pulp and this edible weight has been used in calculating the values given. Where the size of a product varies greatly – for example, a pawpaw or custard apple, values are given for 100g.

Background to effective weight loss

Australians are getting fatter. Everyone is looking for something to blame, but it's hard to go past the fact that we move less and eat more. The health guidelines we really need are just the opposite: move more and eat less. Of course, it's a bit more complicated because we need to remember there is a genetic effect and we also need to eat more of some foods that are currently under-represented in our diet – especially vegetables.

Eating less really refers to the need to reduce our intake of kilojoules and this book aims to make that as painless as possible by increasing the intake of filling foods rich in dietary fibre and leaving in the fuel foods which will provide the energy for exercise.

Compared with earlier generations, we are much less active. The general pace of life means we take every shortcut possible. We drive distances we would once have walked, we have remote control devices, we use spray and wipe cleaners instead of old-fashioned elbow grease and many of us spend long hours sitting in front of TV and computer screens.

The evidence also shows we eat more, but not of everything. We eat fewer vegetables, eat less fruit, fewer wholegrains and even less bread. But we eat more snack foods (chips, crisps, 'health'bars', confectionery), more soft drinks, more fast foods and take away meals and more rich sauces (many used on foods like pasta). We also eat out more and restaurant meals tend to have higher levels of fat than the same foods cooked in the home kitchen. Many restaurants also charge extra for vegetables, so most people tend to do without them.

Over the years, the public has blamed different factors for increasing weight. We used to blame sugar, then all carbohydrates, then fat and now it's again fashionable to blame all carbohydrates.

There is ample evidence from many studies around the world that a high fat intake is most closely correlated with body fat. Those who eat a lot of fat have much higher levels of obesity than those whose diet is low in fat. In Asian countries where the diet was once very high in carbohydrate (usually as rice) with little fat, obesity was almost unknown. As rice consumption has fallen and fat intake has increased, obesity (and diabetes) have risen to disastrous levels.

The solution to the problem of fats causing obesity is not to simply decrease all fat. Some fats are essential for good health, and are especially important in the structure of the brain and of the membranes around every cell. Small quantities of essential fats should form part of all healthy diets.

For some years, health authorities have recommended that we eat less fat and more vegetables, fruits and products made from grains (preferably wholegrains). Some popular diets cite the increasing incidence of obesity as proving that advice to eat less fat doesn't work. In fact, surveys show that few people have really followed the health recommendations. Consumption of fruits, vegetables and wholegrains continues to fall while overall fat consumption remains high.

Fat-reduced processed foods have introduced a complication. Products such as reduced-fat biscuits, snacks, chocolates, ice creams and dairy desserts, yoghurt, dressings and sauces may contain less fat than their regular counterparts, but many have been padded out with extra sugar or refined starches. So even though they have less fat, their kilojoule level is not necessarily reduced. Studies also show that when a label says 'reduced-fat' or 'low fat', most people choose a larger serve or consume the product more often. With some products, when manufacturers release a reduced-fat version, they also bring out a super rich product with even more fat than usual. Fat-reduced ice creams have proliferated, but have been accompanied by extra rich ice cream.

Serving sizes are important. In a healthy balanced diet, nothing needs to be forbidden, but most people require only small quantities of foods that provide concentrated kilojoules.

Serving sizes for many foods have increased. For example, soft drinks once came in 250mL containers. These were replaced by 370mL cans and now 600mL bottles of soft drink are sold as an individual serve. Potato crisps have gone the same way, increasing from 28g to 50g and now to 100g or 200g/packet. Biscuits come in smaller packets, but the idea is to eat the lot rather than take one and place the rest in the biscuit container. Even the humble hamburger has grown – in size, fat and kilojoules. Hamburgers in the 1970s averaged 17g of fat, whereas modern fast food burgers generally have one and a half to twice that much. Part of the reason is the larger size.

Food labels list the nutrition information in a product per 100g and also per serve. The serve size is left to the manufacturer's discretion, and may be different from what the average consumer would eat. So always check that the serving size recommended is similar to what you would consume.

The principles of successful weight loss are to:

- move more (exercise is vital to burn kilojoules and also helps keep the appetite in tune with what the body needs);
- remember that kilojoules count, (which is why it is important to reduce fats and also sugars and refined starchy fillers);
- understand what is in foods. We've included fat and carbohydrate ratings in this edition, as well as kilojoules, fat and fibre content;
- find a healthy eating pattern you can stick to for life. It needs to be rich in essential nutrients and satisfying. Fibre remains the

best way to judge whether a food is filling – it's still nature's obstacle to overeating!

Too much fat

The worst fats are saturated fats which occur naturally in animal products and increase when we consume many foods made from vegetable oils processed in such a way that their saturated fats increase. The process of hydrogenating vegetable oils for processed foods also produces a trans fat (called elaidic acid), which is worse than saturated fat. Many studies show that saturated fats and this introduced trans fat increase the level of 'bad' low density cholesterol (LDL) in the bloodstream.

Unsaturated fats (found in fish, nuts, avocado, olive and liquid vegetable oils) can lower LDL cholesterol levels. These fats have the same kilojoule count as saturated and processed fats, but a much more favourable health effect.

It makes sense to reduce saturated fat intake by choosing low-fat dairy products, trimmed meat and skinless chicken cuts. But it's also important to avoid foods with hidden fats. Over 40% of our saturated fat now comes from processed vegetable oils used in foods such as biscuits, bars, cakes, crisps, chips, pastries and crumbed or coated foods.

About 35% of our food dollar is now spent on foods prepared outside the home, and these foods usually have more fat than the same food cooked at home. Take mashed potatoes for example. Restaurant chefs pride themselves on their creamy mash. They achieve it by using lots more butter and cream than home cooks usually do. A serving of mashed potato in a restaurant is likely to contain 10 times as much fat as a similar-sized serving prepared at home. Similarly, pasta in restaurants is doused with much more oil than when pasta is cooked in the home kitchen and large commercial containers of cream are also poured into sauces for pasta and other foods.

Almost everyone under-reports their food consumption, with the average person failing to report about 20% of what they eat. Overweight people often under-report their intake by up to 50%, not because they are untruthful, but because they are poor at judging how much they are eating. Most people specifically under-report foods high in fat or sugar.

How much fat and which type?

Breast milk has half its energy coming from fat. This is important for a baby's rapid growth and breast milk also contains essential fatty acids that help the developing brain and retina of the eye.

For the first two years, when children are growing rapidly and often have small appetites, the fats in healthy, nutritious foods such as milk, yoghurt, cheese, eggs, chicken, lean meat, avocado and peanut butter (avoid, if allergies present) are important. These foods continue to play an important role until growth stops and parents should not forbid them. However, it is best not to get children used to eating the fat down the edge of some cuts of meat or to have frequent pastries, chocolates, biscuits, crisps or fried foods. These foods are best kept for parties or special occasions.

Adults need much less fat than children. People in Mediterranean countries eat lots of olive oil and nuts and have high levels of health, but too much of most types of fat causes problems, especially with body weight. This does not mean that adults should avoid all fats, but we should choose 'good' fats – and consume them in moderation. For example, omega 3 fats are essential for brain and nerve cells, play an important part in the membranes around every cell in the body and reduce the risk of sudden death from irregular heart rhythms. There is no benefit—and some potential disadvantages—in trying to cut fats to extremely low levels. Fats also carry flavours and make foods taste good and some fat is essential for the absorption of fat-soluble vitamins and antioxidants. Foods such as extra virgin olive oil, nuts and avocado contain unsaturated fats plus their own antioxidants to help prevent fats oxidising in the arteries and forming plaque and clots.

If you do not need to lose weight, the exact intake of fat is not especially important, but you still need to choose mainly 'good' fats and avoid large quantities of saturated fat.

For those trying to lose body fat, the most important aspect of diet is to reduce overall kilojoules. The easiest way to do this is to:

- keep your intake of fat below about 40g a day, possibly reducing this to 30 grams if you are small and inactive;
- keep your overall kilojoule intake moderate to low by also decreasing alcohol, sugar and refined starches.

When you are keeping fat to low levels, make sure the fats you do choose are 'good' fats. Choose foods that have ✓ or ✓✓.

As this book shows, many typical servings of some foods exceed an entire day's desirable level of fat. In some cases, you can reduce fat by using less fat in a recipe. For others, you will need to eat a smaller than average portion, or share the dish with someone else.

If you are very thin and need to gain some body fat, it is important to increase your intake of foods with 'good' fats. Products such as olive oil, nuts and avocado are ideal.

There is ongoing debate about how much fat people with diabetes should consume, but no dispute that most of the fat should be unsaturated 'good' fat. Some researchers have found greater success in controlling diabetes with a diet containing more monounsaturated fats, but reduced total kilojoules, achieved by taking less sugar and alcohol and also limiting foods high in starch. As for most other people, it is important to avoid foods high in saturated fat and to eat plenty of dietary fibre.

Other factors

Choose fats and sugars by the company they keep. Most fried foods and products such as chocolate and other confectionery, biscuits, pastries, chips, snack foods, meat fat and creamy sauces have little or no essential fat or other important nutrients.

By contrast, fish and other seafoods, olive oil and some other vegetable oils, oats and other grains, green vegetables, avocado, nuts, seeds and lean meat and chicken are sources of essential fats and also provide many other important nutrients. Dairy products are also good sources of many nutrients such as calcium and some B complex vitamins.

More on fat types

Most foods contain a mixture of saturated, monounsaturated or polyunsaturated fats. For example, olive oil contains about 75% monounsaturated fat, 13% polyunsaturated and 12% saturated fat. It is called a monounsaturated fat because that is its predominant type of fat.

Saturated fats have adverse effects on blood cholesterol and high levels are linked with some cancers, including bowel cancer.

Saturated fats were once thought to occur mainly as animal fats. These days, saturated vegetable fats from coconut, palm kernel oil and partially hydrogenated vegetable oils used in processed foods, commercial frying and margarines contribute over 40% of our saturated fat intake. Bottled liquid vegetable oils are 'good' fats but you can no longer trust the words 'vegetable oil' in an ingredient list as representing good nutritional value. A margarine labelled as mono or polyunsaturated has 20 to 30% saturated fats, as well as 50 to 60% of unsaturated fats. The total fat content of butter and margarine is the same.

Polyunsaturated fats are essential for humans. The omega 3 polyunsaturates from fish, linseeds, canola, soy beans and walnuts are especially important. Research suggests omega 3 fats are unlikely to be converted to body fat. For balance within the diet, most people should not cut back on omega 3 fats.

The omega 6 polyunsaturates are also important. They are found in foods such as oats, walnuts and soy beans, and in a concentrated form in corn, safflower, sunflower seeds vegetable oils, margarines and mayonnaise. Omega 6 polyunsaturated fats can reduce blood cholesterol effectively, but in animals they are linked with tumours, especially mammary tumours. There has not been any link established between these fats and breast cancer in humans, but they can give rise to reactive chemicals called 'free radicals' which are implicated in heart disease, cancer and ageing. No human population ever consumed large quantities of polyunsaturated fats before food technology made it possible. With these fats, remember that a small quantity is essential, but more is not better.

Too much of the omega 6 fats also prevents the body converting plant omega 3 fats into the same valuable kind as are found in fish and seafood.

Monounsaturated fats are found in olive, macadamia, canola and avocado oils and in most nuts. They are also the predominant type of fat in chicken. Extra virgin olive oil and some macadamia and canola oils are made by cold-pressing without heat or chemical solvents. This allows valuable antioxidants to remain in the oil. Whether it is the type of fat or the high levels of antioxidants in olive oil (or the fact that it is used with vegetables) that makes it so valuable is not clear, but those whose major dietary fat is olive oil have low levels of heart disease and also breast and bowel cancers. Most canola oils are extracted with a chemical solvent, and although canola has an excellent balance of fatty acids, including some of the valuable omega 3s, it does not offer the range of antioxidants found in extra virgin olive oil.

Cholesterol is not included in this book, as it can be a red herring. People who have high levels of blood cholesterol make excessive amounts of cholesterol when they eat saturated fats. The cholesterol content of foods has much less effect on blood cholesterol levels. Cutting back on foods containing saturated fats is much more useful.

Dietary fibre

Just as there are many vitamins and minerals which we need for good health, so there are different types of dietary fibre which have varying degrees of value. For example, soluble fibres like pectin in fruits and vegetable gums can help reduce cholesterol more than insoluble fibre in wheat bran. Both soluble and insoluble fibre are valuable to keep bowel cells healthy, prevent constipation and reduce the risk of bowel cancer. Just as we need the full range of vitamins, so we many different types of fibre.

Dietary fibre helps regulate the gastrointestinal tract. Increasing dietary fibre to 30-40 grams a day will usually prevent or cure constipation and decrease the risk of bowel cancer and diverticular disease. More fibre (but not unprocessed bran) also helps those with irritable bowel syndrome.

For good health, try to eat a variety of fruits, vegetables, cereals and grains, breads, legumes, seeds and nuts to provide many types of dietary fibre as well as a wealth of other nutrients. Most people fail to eat enough fibre because they are so full of fatty, sugary and salty foods that they have no room for high fibre foods.

There is no benefit—and some potential problems with excessive flatulence—if you eat more than 50 to 60g of fibre/day. There is also a possibility that you may absorb less of the minerals from foods if you consume too much fibre, especially from large quantities of unprocessed bran.

Carbohydrate and body weight

Carbohydrates are the body's major source of fuel. Low carb diets 'work' only if they are low in total kilojoules. Some popular diets cut all carbs and achieve a fast initial weight loss. Much of this is water, although a couple of small studies show that low-carb dieters may lose more weight over the first few months of a diet compared with more conventional low fat diets. By 12 months, there is no difference in weight loss between the two diets.

Many foods high in sugar or refined starches (biscuits, cakes, donuts, confectionery, most desserts, soft drinks, savoury snacks) have few nutrients. Eat these foods only occasionally or in small quantities. By contrast, carbohydrate foods such as fruit, potatoes, sweet corn, peas, beans and lentils, wholegrain breads and cereals and reduced fat milk and yoghurt are rich sources of important nutrients and have a low GI. There is no need to cut back on these worthwhile carbohydrate foods

Warning

This book is brief and does not consider all aspects of diet. The healthiest diets include a wide variety of foods, especially a diverse range of plant-based foods.

Acknowledgment

Some of the figures used directly or in calculating values for recipes have been taken from Nutritional Values of Australian Foods (Australian Government Publishing Service). Some of the valuable analytical work for these figures and for my own calculations was provided by Associate Professor H. Greenfield and Professor R.B.H. Wills and others at the University of New South Wales. I thank AGPS and Professor Greenfield for permission to use these.

Food	Fibre g	Fat g	Fat Rating	Energy kJ	Carb Rating
Abalone, grilled, 100g	0	1.0	✓✓	470	
Aduki beans, cooked, 1 cup, 190g	10.5	0.5		1000	✓✓
Aduki beans, dried, 100g	11.0	0.5		1160	✓✓
Agar, (seaweed), raw, 2 tbsp, 10g	0	0		10	
Agar, dried, 10g	1.0	0		130	
Aioli, 1 tbsp, 20g	0	16.0	✓	610	
Aioli, Neil Perry, 1 tbsp, 20g	0	10.0	✓	405	
Aktavite, 3 level teaspoons, 15g	0	1.5	×	235	
Alfalfa sprouts, 1/6 punnet, 30g	0.5	0		50	
All-Bran Fruit 'n Oats, ½ cup, 50g	9.0	2.0	✓✓	700	✓✓
All-bran, ¾ cup, 50g	14.0	2.5	✓✓	550	✓✓
Almond bread, baked, 4 small pieces, 22g	0.5	1.5	✓	220	×
Almond macaroons, home-made, 1	1.0	6.0	×	540	×
Almonds, 50 g	4.5	28.0	✓✓	1240	
Almonds, flaked, 1 tbsp, 8g	0.5	4.5	✓✓	200	
Almonds, slivered, ½ cup, 60g	5.5	33.5	✓✓	1490	
Almonds, weighed in shells, 100g	5.0	20.5	✓✓	935	
Almonds, whole, 20 nuts	3.5	11.5	✓✓	625	
Amaranth leaves, 50g	1.0	0		40	
Anchovy, average fillet, 7g	0	0.5	✓	55	
Angel cake, 1/10 20cm cake	0.5	0		760	××
Antipasto, mixed (delicatessen), ½ cup	2.5	15.0	✓	990	✓
Ants, green tree, 5g	0	0		25	
Ants, honey, 5g	0	0		55	
Anzac biscuits, commercial, 1	0.5	4.5	××	370	××
Anzac biscuits, home-made, 1	0.5	3.0	××	250	××
Apple & walnut scroll bun, 1, 90g	2.5	7.0	×	1015	✓
Apple cider, alcoholic, dry, 250 mL	0	0		400	
Apple cider, alcoholic, sweet, 250 mL	0	0		560	×
Apple cider, non alcoholic, 250 mL	0	0		415	×
Apple crumble, average serve	2.5	17.0	×	1675	×

Food	Fibre g	Fat g	Fat Rating	Energy kJ	Carb Rating
Apple cucumber, 1/4 medium, 80g	1.0	0		25	
Apple flan, French, home made, 1/6 20 cm flan	4.5	18.5	××	1895	××
Apple juice concentrate, 1 tbsp, 20 mL	0	0		140	
Apple juice drink, 35% juice, 250 mL	0	0		425	×
Apple juice, carbonated, 250 mL	0	0		435	×
Apple juice, no sugar, 250 mL	0	0		440	✓✓
Apple pie, double crust, 1/6 pie	2.5	21.0	××	1515	××
Apple pie, frozen, 1/6 of pie, 135g	2.0	18.5	××	1365	××
Apple pie, home-made, 1/6 23 cm pie	5.5	28.0	××	2520	××
Apple pie, McDonalds, 1	1.5	18.5	××	1250	××
Apple strudel, average serve	7.0	29.0	××	2475	××
Apple strudel, home-made, 1/10 strudel	4.0	23.0	××	1800	××
Apple strudel, puff pastry, average serve	4.0	34.0	××	2055	××
Apple tea cake, 1/6 18 cm cake	3.0	10.0	××	1060	××
Apple, 1 large, cored, 200g	4.0	0		400	✓✓
Apple, 1 medium, cored and peeled, 135g	2.5	0		280	✓✓
Apple, 1 medium, cored, 150g	3.0	0		310	✓✓
Apple, 1 small, cored, 100g	2.0	0		200	✓✓
Apple, canned pie pack, 1 cup, 240g	3.0	0		400	✓✓
Apple, canned pieces, no sugar, 1 cup, 220g	3.0	0		420	✓✓
Apple, canned slices, with syrup, 1 cup, 250g	2.5	0		700	✓
Apple, dried, 10 rings, 35g	2.5	0		355	✓✓
Apple, snack pack, 135g	4.0	0		590	✓✓
Apple, stewed, 1 cup	3.5	0		900	✓✓
Apple, stuffed, baked, 1	4.5	0.5	×	640	✓✓
Applesauce, 1 tbsp	0	0		45	
Applesauce, home-made, 1 tbsp	0	0		55	✓
Apricot bread, dry baked, 28g	0.5	0.5	✓	455	×
Apricot delight bar, 6 small squares, 45g	3.0	3.0	×	525	×
Apricot juice drink, 35% juice, 250 mL	1.0	0		575	×
Apricot nectar, 50% juice, 250 mL	1.5	0		665	✓

Food	Fibre g	Fat g	Fat Rating	Energy kJ	Carb Rating
Apricot, 1 large, 70g	1.5	0		110	✓✓
Apricot, canned in juice, drained, 6 halves	2.5	0		215	✓
Apricot, canned in syrup, ½ cup	2.5	0		330	✗
Apricot, canned in syrup, drained, 6 halves	2.5	0		265	✗
Apricot, canned in water, no sugar, 6 halves	2.0	0		125	✓✓
Apricot, canned, pie pack, 1 cup, 225g	3.5	0		225	✓✓
Apricot, canned, snack pack, 140g	2.5	0		320	✓
Apricot, canned, snack pack, Lite, 140g	2.5	0		295	✓✓
Apricot, dried, 1 cup, 150g	9.0	0		820	✓✓
Apricot, dried, 3 whole, 50g	4.5	0		410	✓✓
Apricot, dried, 6 large halves, 35g	3.0	0		285	✓✓
Apricot, dried, 6 small halves, 25g	2.5	0		205	✓✓
Armenian nutmeg cake, 1/8 29 cm cake	5.0	22.0	✗✗	1775	✗✗
Arrowroot, 1 tbsp, 10g	0	0		145	
Artichoke, canned, 1 heart, 50g	1.5	0		35	
Artichoke, globe, 1 medium	1.5	0		105	
Artichoke, Jerusalem, 100g	3.0	0		100	
Artichoke, marinated in oil, 1 large	1.5	3.5	✓✓	295	
Asia at home, stir-fry noodles, 100g	0.5	1.0	✓	740	✓
Asia at home, sweet chilli sauce, 2 tbsp	0	0		120	
Asia at home, udon noodles, 100g	0.5	0.5		580	✓
Asparagus, canned, drained, 8 spears	4.0	0		70	
Asparagus, fresh, 8 thin or 4 thick spears, 120g	2.0	0		85	
Atlantic salmon, fresh, grilled, 150g	0	4.0	✓✓	765	
Aubergine, baby, 4, 65g	1.5	0		50	
Aubergine, fried in minimum oil, 100g	2.5	8.0	✓✓	375	
Aubergine, fried in olive oil, 100g	2.5	25.0	✓✓	1000	
Aubergine, grilled, 3 slices, 90g	2.5	0		65	
Aubergine, marinated in oil, 100g	2.5	25.0	✓✓	1000	
Aubergine, raw, 100g	2.5	0		75	
Avocado oil, 1 tbsp	0	20.0	✓✓	740	

Food	Fibre g	Fat g	Fat Rating	Energy kJ	Carb Rating
Avocado, ½ large, 110g	1.5	25.0	✓✓	965	
Avocado, ½ small, flesh, 80 g	1.0	18.0	✓✓	705	
Avocado, cocktail size, 1, 30g	0.5	7.0	✓✓	265	
Baba ghannouj (eggplant dip), average serve, 60g	5.5	12.0	✓✓	610	
Baba, rum (cake), average serve	1.5	8.5	××	1370	××
Babaco, 100g	1.0	0		80	
Baby rusks, each, 8g	0	0.5		120	
Baby yoghurt desserts, 110g jar	0	1.5	×	345	
Bacon bits, 2 teaspoons, 8g	0	1.5	×	125	
Bacon, fried & 2 fried eggs	0	32.0	×	1660	
Bacon, lean grilled & 2 poached eggs	0	14.5	×	1010	
Bacon, middle, fried, 1 rasher, 35g	0	10.5	×	545	
Bacon, middle, fried, trimmed, 1 rasher, 28g	0	3.0	×	265	
Bacon, middle, grilled, 1 rasher, 32g	0	7.0	×	430	
Bacon, middle, grilled, trimmed, 1 rasher, 26g	0	3.0	×	260	
Bacon, middle, raw, trimmed, 100g	0	5.5	×	570	
Bagel crisps, 5, 50g	0.5	7.5	×	910	✓
Bagel, average, 90g	2.0	1.5	✓	1035	✓
Bagel/chicken & avocado	5.0	37.0	✓	2780	✓
Bagel/eggplant, sundried tomato, pesto, cheese	6.0	36.0	×	2380	✓
Bagel/goats cheese & rocket	4.0	12.0	×	1580	✓
Bagel/smoked salmon, cream cheese	4.0	11.0	×	1590	✓
Baguette, French bread, 1/3 medium, 75g	4.0	2.0	×	860	✓
Baked beans, canned, ½ can, 220g	10.5	1.0	✓	630	✓✓
Bakers cheese, 100g	0	2.5	×	390	
Bakers chips, 30g	0.5	4.5	✓	575	✓
Baklava, commercial, 100g	2.0	19.5	××	1540	××
Baklava, home-made, average piece	2.0	25.0	××	1870	××
Baklava, purchased, small piece, 50g	2.0	18.5	××	1040	××
Balance oat bran flakes, 1 cup, 30g	3.5	1.0	✓	480	✓✓

Food	Fibre g	Fat g	Fat Rating	Energy kJ	Carb Rating
Bamboo shoots, canned, 1 cup, 140g	2.5	0		45	
Banana chips, sweetened, 20 chips, 22g	1.0	0		245	✗
Banana fritters, 1	3.0	29.0	✗✗	1840	
Banana smoothie, 1	2.0	10.0	✗	1230	✓✓
Banana smoothie, fat-reduced, 1	2.0	4.0	✗	1100	✓✓
Banana split, average	4.0	32.0	✗	2575	✗
Banana, 1 large, weighed with skin, 220g	3.0	0.5		500	✓✓
Banana, 1 small, weighed with skin, 120g	2.0	0		270	✓✓
Banana, dried, 1	3.0	0		450	✓✓
Banana, sugar, 1, weighed with skin, 140g	3.0	0		355	✓✓
Barbecue pork, Chinese, 1 piece, 120g	0	18.0	✗	1200	
Barbecue sauce, 1 tbsp	0	0		145	
Barbecue sauce, fast food portion pack, 1	0	0.5		180	✗
Barley bran, 1 tbsp, 10g	1.5	0.5		130	✓✓
Barley, cooked, 1 cup, 180g	6.5	1.5	✓	800	✓✓
Barley, quick cook, 100g	13.0	3.0	✓	1275	✓✓
Barley, raw, ½ cup, 105g	9.5	2.5	✓	1330	✓✓
Basil, fresh, 1 cup, 30g	1.5	0		35	
Bavarois, average serve	0	21.0	✗	1100	✗✗
Bean curd, fried, 100g	6.5	11.0	✗	690	
Bean soup, 1 large bowl, 430g	7.0	12.0	✓✓	800	✓✓
Bean sprouts, mung, ½ cup, 45g	1.5	0		40	
Bean stew, average serve	10.0	18.0	✗	1200	✓✓
Beans 'n' corn, canned, 100g	n/a	1.0	✓	405	✓✓
Beans, baked with sausages, canned, 1 cup 220g	8.5	4.0	✗	1065	✓✓
Beans, baked, canned, 1 cup, 220g	9.0	1.0	✓	760	✓✓
Beans, baked, canned, vegetarian, 1 cup, 220g	9.0	1.5	✓	845	✓✓
Beans, black gram, cooked, 1 cup, 190g	11.0	1.0	✓	720	✓✓
Beans, black gram, raw, 100g	18.0	1.5	✓	1170	✓✓
Beans, blackeye, canned, drained, 100g	6.0	0.5		515	✓✓

Food	Fibre g	Fat g	Fat Rating	Energy kJ	Carb Rating
Beans, blackeye, cooked, 1 cup, 185g	6.5	1.5	✓	915	✓✓
Beans, blackeye, dried, ½ cup, 100g	8.0	1.5	✓	1325	✓✓
Beans, borlotti, canned, drained, 100g	6.5	0.5		470	✓✓
Beans, broad, fresh, ½ cup, 60g	2.5	0		105	✓
Beans, broad, frozen, ½ cup cooked, 80g	7.0	0		245	✓
Beans, butter, fresh, ½ cup cooked, 70g	2.0	0		55	✓
Beans, canned, three bean mix, 1 cup, 185g	11.5	0.5		665	✓✓
Beans, cannellini, canned, 1 cup, 190g	12.0	1.0	✓	585	✓✓
Beans, cannellini, dried, 100g	23.0	1.5	✓	1220	✓✓
Beans, French/green, fresh or frozen, 100g	2.5	0		85	
Beans, haricot, cooked, 180g	16.0	1.5	✓	680	✓✓
Beans, haricot, dried, 100g	18.5	2.0	✓	1050	✓✓
Beans, kidney, canned, ½ cup, 95g	6.0	0.5		340	✓✓
Beans, kidney, cooked, 1 cup, 185g	20.0	0.5		890	✓✓
Beans, kidney, dried, ½ cup, 95g	10.5	0.5		455	✓✓
Beans, Lima, canned, drained, 1 cup, 220g	10.0	1.0	✓	720	✓✓
Beans, Lima, cooked, 1 cup, 180g	8.5	1.0	✓	785	✓✓
Beans, Lima, dried, uncooked, ½ cup, 90g	18.0	1.5	✓	1110	✓✓
Beans, Mexican chilli, canned, 210g	11.0	1.0	✓	670	✓✓
Beans, mixed, canned, drained, 1 cup, 220g	9.5	2.0	✓	495	✓✓
Beans, mung beans, cooked, 1 cup, 200g	5.0	0.5		390	✓✓
Beans, mung, dry, 100g	14.0	1.0	✓	1190	✓✓
Beans, pinto beans, dry, ½ cup, 95g	23.0	1.0	✓	1350	✓✓
Beans, pinto, cooked, 1 cup, 180g	15.5	1.5	✓	1050	✓✓
Beans, purple, cooked, ½ cup, 70g	3.0	0		85	
Beans, runner, 100g	2.5	0		85	
Beans, snake, 100g	3.0	0		95	
Beans, soy, canned, drained, 1 cup, 200g	8.5	2.0	✓✓	790	✓✓
Beans, soy, cooked, 1 cup, 200g	14.5	14.5	✓✓	1080	✓✓
Beans, soy, dry, ½ cup, 100g	20.0	20.0	✓✓	1420	✓✓
Bearnaise sauce, 2 tbsps	0	18.0	✗✗	715	

Food	Fibre g	Fat g	Fat Rating	Energy kJ	Carb Rating
Bechamel sauce, 2 tbsps	0	10.0	××	465	
Beef cake, Vietnamese, average serve	0.5	7.0	×	860	
Beef rissoles with honey, 2, 150g	0	23.0	××	1190	
Beef satay, 2 skewers	7.0	25.0	×	1500	
Beef sausage, 1, 110g	0	22.0	××	915	
Beef sausage, thin, grilled, 1, 80g	0	15.0	××	855	
Beef tongue, cooked, 100g	0	25.0	×	1290	
Beef, big burger patties, frozen, 1 patty, 125g	1.0	12.5	×	825	
Beef, black bean sauce, 150g	3.0	11.0	×	680	✓
Beef, blade steak, raw, lean & fat, 100g	0	11.0	×	745	
Beef, blade steak, raw, lean only, 100g	0	6.0	×	580	
Beef, Bolognaise sauce, average serve, 160g	2.0	17.5	×	965	
Beef, braised steak & onion, 1 medium can, 340g	5.5	40.5	×	2435	
Beef, brisket (corned beef), boiled, lean only, 100g	0	10.0	×	890	
Beef, brisket, boiled, lean & fat, 100g,	0	23.5	×	1300	
Beef, casserole, average serve, 250g	2.0	18.0	×	1260	
Beef, chilli con carne, average serve	5.3	24.0	×	1650	✓
Beef, chow mein, average serve, 250g	1.5	15.0	×	1430	
Beef, chuck steak, raw, lean only, 100g	0	3.0	×	455	
Beef, chuck steak, raw, trimmed, 100g	0	6.0	×	560	
Beef, consomme, 1 cup, 250 mL	0	0		135	
Beef, corned & cereal, canned, 100g	1.5	13.5	×	825	×
Beef, corned silverside, 60g	0	1.5	×	250	
Beef, corned, canned, 100g	0	11.0	×	805	
Beef, curry, Indian, average serve, 250g	1.0	16.5	×	1440	
Beef, curry, Thai (coconut milk), average serve	1.5	44.0	×	2580	
Beef, fillet steak, grilled, trimmed, 100g	0	10.0	×	880	
Beef, fillet steak, raw, lean, 100g	0	7.5	×	630	
Beef, goulash, average serve	2.5	20.0	×	1840	

Food	Fibre g	Fat g	Fat Rating	Energy kJ	Carb Rating
Beef, hamburger patties, frozen, 1 thin patty, 50g	0.5	10.0	×	550	
Beef, hamburger patties, home-made, 1 patty	0.5	24.0	×	1540	
Beef, koftas, average serve, 175g	1.5	48.0	×	2570	
Beef, meatballs, average serve, 230g	1.5	19.0	×	1625	
Beef, meatloaf, 1 slice	1.0	28.0	×	2140	
Beef, mince, 90% fat-free, raw, 100gt	0	10.0	×	685	
Beef, mince, extra lean, 95% fat free, raw, 100g	0	5.0	×	540	
Beef, mince, raw, 100g	0	11.0	×	740	
Beef, moussaka, average serve	2.0	26.0	×	1500	✓
Beef, oyster sauce, average serve	0.5	19.0	×	1245	
Beef, pepper steak, fried, 200g	0	26.0	×	1800	
Beef, pie, home-made, average serve	1.5	36.0	××	2500	××
Beef, rib eye, grilled, lean & fat, 150g	0	24.0	×	1600	
Beef, rib eye, grilled, trimmed, small steak, 130g	0	10.0	×	1075	
Beef, rissoles, 2, 340g	3.5	31.0	××	2780	×
Beef, round steak, raw, lean & fat, 100g	0	9.0	×	675	
Beef, round steak, raw, trimmed, 100g	0	6.5	×	590	
Beef, rump steak, grilled, lean, 150g	0	10.0	×	1200	
Beef, rump steak, raw, trimmed, 140g	0	8.5	×	850	
Beef, rump, grilled, extra lean, 150g	0	7.0	×	910	
Beef, rump, raw, extra lean, 140g	0	5.5g	×	700	
Beef, silverside, baked, lean & fat, 2 slices, 85g	0	8.5	×	825	
Beef, silverside, baked, trimmed, 2 slices, 80g	0	3.5	×	595	
Beef, sirloin steak, grilled, lean & fat, 1 steak, 180g	0	34.0	×	2070	
Beef, sirloin steak, grilled, trimmed, 1 steak, 140g	0	16.0	×	1265	
Beef, skirt steak, raw, lean & fat, 100g	0	3.5	×	515	
Beef, skirt steak, raw, lean only, 100g	0	2.5	×	470	
Beef, steak Diane, medium fillet	0	29.0	×	1650	

Food	Fibre g	Fat g	Fat Rating	Energy kJ	Carb Rating
Beef, stroganoff, average serve	2.5	48.0	×	2620	×
Beef, teriyaki, 1 cup	0	12.5	×	1330	
Beef, topside roast, 2 slices, lean & fat, 90g	0	9.0	×	720	
Beef, topside roast, 2 slices, lean only, 80g	0	4.0	×	570	
Beef, topside, raw, lean, 100g	0	4.5	×	525	
Beef, Wellington, average serve, 330g	1.0	38.0	×	2750	××
Beer, ale (4.1% alc.), 1 middie, 280 mL	0	0		405	
Beer, bitter/draught (3.7% alc.), middie, 280 mL	0	0		415	
Beer, bitter/draught (3.7% alc.), middie, 280 mL	0	0		415	
Beer, lager (4.0% alc.), 1 can, 370 mL	0	0		570	
Beer, low alcohol (0.7% alc.), 1 can, 370 mL	0	0		160	
Beer, reduced alcohol (2.1% alc.), 1 can, 370 mL	0	0		390	
Beer, regular (3.8% alc.), 1 can, 370 mL	0	0		555	
Beetroot, canned, 5 slices, 100g	2.5	0		175	✓
Beetroot, cooked, 1 medium, 100g	2.5	0		175	✓
Beetroot, raw, grated, 30g	1.0	0		50	✓
Belgian endive, 1 head, 60g	0.5	0		30	
Berliner sausage, 100g	1.0	18.0	××	945	
Besan (chick pea flour), 100g	13.5	5.5	✓	1330	✓✓
Bhuja mix snack, 50g	3.5	18.5	✓	1140	✓
Big Mac, 1	5.0	25.0	×	2010	✓
Biscotti, 2 pieces, 10g	0.5	1.5	✓	170	×
Biscuits, Anzac, commercial, 1	0.5	4.5	×	370	××
Biscuits, Anzac, home-made, 1	0.5	3.0	×	250	××
Biscuits, brandy snaps (cream-filled), 1	0	11.5	××	715	××
Biscuits, chocolate chip, 2, 23g	0.5	6.0	××	450	××
Biscuits, chocolate coated, 1, 15g	0	3.5	××	300	××
Biscuits, chocolate, 2, 20g	0.5	3.5	××	365	××
Biscuits, crackers, cheese, 4 small, 16g	0.5	4.0	××	315	××

Food	Fibre g	Fat g	Fat Rating	Energy kJ	Carb Rating
Biscuits, crackers, flaky texture, 6 small, 24g	0.5	4.0	××	415	××
Biscuits, cream & jam filled, 1, 21g	0.5	4.5	××	400	××
Biscuits, cream filled, 1, 15g	0	3.5	××	305	××
Biscuits, cream wafer type, 2, 11g	0	3.0	××	220	××
Biscuits, dried fruit filling, 2, 35g	1.0	3.0	××	470	××
Biscuits, fruit & nut, 2, 25g	0.5	6.5	××	505	××
Biscuits, fruitables, banana, 1, 25g	1.5	5.0	×	410	×
Biscuits, fruitables, peach, 1, 25g	2.0	1.5	×	400	×
Biscuits, fruitables, sultana, 1, 25g	1.5	4.5	×	400	×
Biscuits, ginger 2, 25g	0.5	3.5	××	575	××
Biscuits, gluten-free Chocolate Blitz, 1	1.5	3.5	×	350	××
Biscuits, gluten-free strawberry slice, 1, 50g	3.0	1.5	×	630	××
Biscuits, home-made chocolate, 1	1.0	17.0	××	1330	××
Biscuits, home-made peanut and honey, 1	2.0	19.0	××	1220	××
Biscuits, home-made, plain, 1	0.5	9.0	××	775	××
Biscuits, iced, 2, 28g	0.5	3.5	××	490	××
Biscuits, jam, 2, 27g	0.5	4.5	××	485	××
Biscuits, ladyfingers, 2, 22g	0	2.0	××	335	××
Biscuits, lattice, 2, 20g	0.5	5.5	××	440	××
Biscuits, macaroons, home-made, 1	1.0	4.0	××	485	×
Biscuits, marshmallow & chocolate, 1, 20g	0	4.0	××	360	××
Biscuits, marshmallow topped, 2, 35g	0.5	5.5	××	590	××
Biscuits, plain sweet, 2, 20g	0.5	3.5	××	375	××
Biscuits, polyunsaturated cookies, 1 17g	0.5	3.5	✓	305	××
Biscuits, Sao, 3, 27g	1.0	4.0	××	470	××
Biscuits, see also Crackers					
Biscuits, shortbread, commercial, 2, 35g	0.5	8.5	××	720	××
Biscuits, shortbread, home-made, 30g	0.5	6.5	××	550	××
Biscuits, shortbread, Unibic, 1, 15g	0	2.0	××	285	×
Biscuits, Tim Tams, 1, 19g	0	5.5	××	400	××
Biscuits, wattleseed & lemon myrtle, 2 , 16g	n/a	1.5	×	355	××

Food	Fibre g	Fat g	Fat Rating	Energy kJ	Carb Rating
Biscuits, wheatmeal, 2, 16g	1.0	3.0	✗	300	✗
Bitter melon (balsam pear or foo gwa)	1.5	0		20	
Black forest cake, small slice, 85g	0.5	16.5	✗✗	1225	✗✗
Black forest cherry cake, 1/10 average cake	2.0	34.0	✗✗	2400	✗✗
Black pudding (sausage), grilled, 100g	2.0	23.5	✗✗	1310	
Blackberries, ½ punnet, 100g	6.5	0		105	
Blackberries, canned in syrup, ½ cup	6.5	0		315	✗
Blackberries, frozen, 1 cup, 150g	10.0	0		155	
Blackfish, 150g	0	2.0	✓	375	
Blancmange, average serve	0	5.0	✗	620	✗
Blancmange, chocolate, average serve	0	10	✗	1050	✗✗
Blini, 3 small	1.0	12.0	✗	950	
Bloody Mary	0	0		520	
Blue eye fish, grilled, 150g	0	2.0	✓✓	640	
Blueberries, ½ punnet, 100g	4.0	0		235	
Blueberries, frozen, 100g	3.5	0		210	
Boboli pizza crust, 1, 112g	3.0	5.0	✓	1245	✓
Bogong moths, 3, 25g	0	5.5	✓	315	
Bolognaise sauce, average serve, 160g	2.0	17.5	✗✗	965	
Bombay savoury snack mix, 25g	1.5	8.0	✗✗	525	✗✗
Bombe Alaska, 1/6 average cake	1.0	21.0	✗✗	1900	✗✗
Bonox, 1 tsp	0	0		20	
Borsch, 1 large bowl	9.0	9.0	✗	840	
Bouillabaisse, 1 large bowl	2.0	12.0	✓✓	1500	
Bounty bar, 1, 50g	2.5	13.0	✗✗	990	✗✗
Boysenberries, canned in syrup, ½ cup	5.5	0		460	✗
Boysenberries, frozen, 1 cup, 130g	5.0	0.5		275	✓✓
Boysenberries, raw, 100g	7.0	0.5		205	✓✓
Braised steak & onion, 1 medium can, 340g	5.5	40.5	✗	2435	
Bran Bix, 2, 30g	6.5	1.0	✓	355	✓✓
Bran buds, ½ cup, 50g	14.0	1.5	✓	580	✓✓

Food	Fibre g	Fat g	Fat Rating	Energy kJ	Carb Rating
Bran muffins, cake-type, 1, 65g	2.0	5.0	×	530	×
Bran, barley, cereal, 10g	1.5	0.5		130	✓✓
Bran, multi bran cereal, ½ cup, 55g	11.5	7.0	✓	955	✓✓
Bran, oat, crunchy, ½ cup, 50g	7.0	2.5	✓	720	✓✓
Bran, oat, raw, ¼ cup, 35g	6.0	3.0	✓	520	✓✓
Bran, processed, ½ cup, 45g	13.0	1.0	✓	495	✓✓
Bran, rice, crunchy 1 tbsp, 10g	2.5	2.0	✓	175	✓✓
Bran, rice, crunchy, ½ cup, 55g	14.0	11.0	✓	975	✓✓
Bran, wheat, unprocessed, 2 tbsp, 12g	5.5	0.5		80	✓✓
Brandy Alexander, 90 mL	0	15.0	××	1175	
Brandy butter, 1 ½ tbsp	0	7.5	××	615	
Brandy, 1 nip, 30 mL	0	0		255	
Branflakes with fruit, 1 cup, 60g	7.5	1.5	✓	780	✓✓
Branflakes, 1 cup, 40g	7.0	1.0	✓	570	✓✓
Brawn, 1 slice, 60g	0	10.0	×	545	
Brazil nuts, 50g	4.5	34.0	✓✓	1410	
Bread & butter custard, average serve	1.5	18.0	×	1530	×
Bread pudding, average serve, 110g	3.0	9.5	×	1365	×
Bread roll, country grain, 1, 65g	3.5	2.0	✓✓	600	✓✓
Bread roll, crusty dinner, 1 small, 35g	1.5	1.0	✓	415	✓
Bread roll, white, average, 60g	2.0	1.5	×	650	✓
Bread roll, wholemeal, average, 60g	3.5	1.5	✓	600	✓
Bread sticks, 3 x 20 cm, 18g	0.5	1.0	✓	300	✓
Bread sticks, 3 x 24 cm, 30g	0.5	1.5	✓	515	✓
Bread UP, DHA, 1 slice, 37g	1.0	1.9	✓	380	✓
Bread, bake at home Turkish, 70g	1.5	3.0	✓	750	✓
Bread, bake at home, dinner rolls, 1, 40g	1.0	1.0	×	450	✓
Bread, bread-maker, 1 slice, 110g	3.0	2.5	✓	1150	✓
Bread, Burgen, Bran & honey, 1 slice, 40g	2.5	2.0	✓	370	✓✓
Bread, Burgen, Oat & Honey, 1 slice, 40g	2.5	2.0	✓	405	✓✓
Bread, Burgen, Soy lin, 1 slice, 40g	2.0	3.0	✓✓	405	✓✓

Food	Fibre g	Fat g	Fat Rating	Energy kJ	Carb Rating
Bread, Burgen, Traditional Rye, 1 slice, 40g	2.0	1.5	✓	370	✓✓
Bread, cape fruit & nut roll, 1, 85g	6.0	6.5	✓✓	1055	✓✓
Bread, cape seed bread, 1 slice, 50g	7.5	2.5	✓✓	565	✓✓
Bread, cape seed roll, 1, 85g	12.5	4.5	✓✓	960	✓✓
Bread, cheese and bacon roll, 1, 100g	2.5	11.0	✗	1230	✓
Bread, cheese and olive roll, 1, 100g	3.0	10.0	✗	1160	✓
Bread, cheese and pineapple roll, 1, 110g	2.5	8.5	✗	1200	✓
Bread, cheese, herb, garlic filled, 1, 165g	6.0	14.5	✗	2395	✓
Bread, cheeseymite scroll, 1, 110g	3.0	11.5	✗	1430	✓
Bread, custard scroll bun, 90g	2.0	7.0	✗	1145	✗
Bread, dark rye, 1 slice, 50g	3.5	1.0	✓	425	✓✓
Bread, fibre increased, 2 slices, 56g	2.5	1.5	✓	545	✓✓
Bread, focaccia, 100g (see also focaccia)	2.5	9.0	✓	1040	✓
Bread, fried, 1 slice, 40g	1.5	12.0	✗✗	840	✓
Bread, fruit loaf, 1 slice, 40g	1.0	2.0	✗	515	✓
Bread, hamburger bun, 1, 60g	2.5	3.0	✗	675	✓
Bread, home sliced, 1 slice, 60g	1.5	1.5	✓	700	✓
Bread, Lavash, 1 slice	1.0	1.0	✓	470	✓
Bread, Lebanese, large, 115g	3.0	2.5	✓	1290	✓
Bread, Lebanese, large, wholemeal, 120g	7.5	2.5	✓	1185	✓✓
Bread, light rye, 1 slice, 30g	1.5	0.5		300	✓
Bread, mixed grain, 1 slice, 28g	1.5	1.0	✓	270	✓✓
Bread, pane di casa, 1 slice, 50g	1.5	1.5	✓	585	✓
Bread, pita, 1 medium, 75g	3.0	1.0	✓	840	✓
Bread, pita, 1 small, 60g	2.5	0.5		675	✓
Bread, pizza roll, 1, 100g	3.0	11.0	✗	1245	✓
Bread, pumpernickel, 1 slice, 50g	3.5	0.5		305	✓✓
Bread, pumpkin, 1 slice, 50g	1.5	2.0	✓	615	✓
Bread, sour dough rye, 1 slice, 60g	3.0	1.0	✓	670	✓✓
Bread, sour dough white, 1 slice, 60g	2.0	1.0	✓	640	✓✓
Bread, sweet apple & walnut scroll, 1, 90g	2.5	7.0	✗	1015	✓

Food	Fibre g	Fat g	Fat Rating	Energy kJ	Carb Rating
Bread, sweet, almond custard scroll, 1, 160g	3.5	24.0	×	2370	×
Bread, sweet, apricot delight roll, 1, 80g	3.5	0.5		920	✓✓
Bread, sweet, caramel scroll, 1, 120g	2.5	6.0	×	1535	×
Bread, sweet, cinnamon scroll, 1, 90g	3.0	3.0	✓	1100	✓
Bread, sweet, coffee & date roll, 1, 85g	3.5	1.0	✓	985	✓
Bread, sweet, finger bun, iced, 1, 85g	2.0	3.0	✓	1130	✓
Bread, sweet, finger bun, no icing, 1, 65g	2.0	3.0	✓	810	✓
Bread, sweet, fruit bun, mini, 1 35g	1.0	1.0	✓	450	✓✓
Bread, sweet, jam scroll with fruit, 1, 120g	3.5	3.0	✓	1560	✓
Bread, toast thickness, 1 slice, 32g	1.0	1.0	×	335	✓
Bread, Vienna, 1 slice, 40g	1.5	1.5	×	445	✓
Bread, Vogels soy & linseed, 1 slice, 38g	4.0	2.5	✓✓	395	✓✓
Bread, white sliced, 1 slice, 32g	1.0	1.0	×	330	✓
Bread, wholemeal, sliced, 32g	2.0	1.0	✓	300	✓
Breadcrumbs, commercial, 1 tbsp, 10g	0.5	0		150	✓
Breadcrumbs, fresh homemade, 2 tbsp, 10g	0.5	0		150	✓
Breadfruit, fresh, ¼ small, 100g	5.0	0		430	✓
Breakfast bars, Be Natural, fruit & nut, 1, 40g	3.0	10.5	✓✓	795	✓✓
Breakfast bars, Be Natural, nut delight, 1, 40g	3.0	14.0	✓✓	895	✓✓
Breakfast bars, Fruit Bake with grains, 1, 40g	2.0	3.5	×	580	✓
Breakfast bars, Fruity Bix, average, 1, 25g	1.5	2.5	×	440	✓
Breakfast bars, Just Right, 1, 33g	2.0	0.5		510	××
Breakfast bars, K-Time, honey nut, 1 33g	0.5	1.0	×	535	××
Breakfast bars, K-Time, mixed berry, 1, 28g	1.0	0.5	×	435	××
Breakfast bars, K-Time, muffin bar, apple, 1, 45g	0.5	4.0	×	720	××
Breakfast bars, K-Time, Twist, 1, 37g	1.0	1.0	×	515	××
Breakfast bars, LCM, chocolate chip, 1, 22g	0	2.5	×	390	××
Breakfast bars, LCM, cornflakes & honey, 1, 22g	0.5	1.0	×	355	××
Breakfast bars, LCM, honey rice bubbles, 1, 22g	0	1.5	×	370	××
Breakfast bars, Oven Baked Muesli Crunch, 1, 50g	2.5	12.0	×	1020	××

Food	Fibre g	Fat g	Fat Rating	Energy kJ	Carb Rating
Breakfast bars, see also muesli bars					
Breakfast bars, Sustain, 1 33g	1.0	0.5		530	××
Breakfast bars, Uncle Toby's Fruit & Nut, 1, 37g	1.5	4.5	✓	615	××
Breakfast bars, Uncle Toby's, average, 1, 37g	2.0	2.0	✓	550	×
Breakfast bars, Uncle Toby's, Lite Start, 1, 37g	2.0	3.0	✓	590	××
Breakfast bars, Uncle Toby's, Sports Plus, 1, 37g	2.0	3.0	✓	610	××
Breakfast bars, Weight Watchers, fruit, 1, 40g	1.5	0.5		480	×
Breakfast, Up and Go soy drink, 285 mL	4.0	4.0	✓	850	✓
Breakfast-on-the-go bar, 1, 36g	2.0	2.0	✓	550	×
Breakfast-on-the-go liquid, 285mL	5.5	4.5	✓	940	✓
Brioche, individual, 1	2.0	10.0	××	1145	×
Broad beans, 1 cup fresh, cooked, 110	6.0	0.5		220	✓
Broad beans, frozen, ½ cup cooked, 75g	5.0	0.5		260	✓
Broad beans, mature, 1 cup cooked, 170g	9.0	0.5		780	✓
Broccoli in cream sauce, frozen, 125g	1.5	3.0	×	240	
Broccoli, average serve, 100g	4.0	0		100	
Broccolini, average serve, 100g	1.5	0		180	
Brownie, chocolate, 1, 100g	1.0	30.0	××	1920	××
Brownies, fudge, 1 small, 40g	0.5	12.0	××	770	××
Bruschetta with tomato, 1 slice	2.0	8.0	✓	650	✓
Bruschetta, 1 slice	1.0	8.0	✓	570	✓
Brussels sprouts, average serve, 5, 100g	3.5	0		105	
Bubble & squeak, average serve, ¾ cup	2.5	4.0	×	450	✓
Buffalo milk, 1 cup, 250 mL	0	17.0	×	1010	✓
Buffalo, roasted, 100g	0	2.0	✓	550	
Bulgur (cracked wheat), raw, ½ cup, 75g	12.0	1.5	✓	940	✓✓
Bulgur, cooked, 1 cup, 250g	10.5	1.0	✓	900	✓✓
Bun finger, iced, 1, 65g	2.0	3.0	✓	1130	×
Bun finger, sugar-glazed, 1, 65g	2.0	3.0	✓	810	✓
Buns, hot cross fruit, home-made, each	1.5	4.0	×	875	✓
Bunya nut, 50g	3.5	0.5		400	✓✓

Food	Fibre g	Fat g	Fat Rating	Energy kJ	Carb Rating
Burgen, see bread					
Burrito tortilla, unfilled, 1, 40g	2.0	3.5	×	545	✓
Burrito wrap, 1, 46g	1.5	4.0	×	605	✓
Burrito, 1	8.0	31.0	×	3600	✓
Burrito, beef filling, 1, 200g	5.0	26.0	×	2280	✓
Butter beans, fresh, ½ cup cooked, 70g	2.0	0		55	✓
Butter cake, 1/8 20 cm cake	1.5	15.0	××	1385	××
Butter sprinkles, 1 tsp	0	0		35	
Butter, 1 tbsp, 20g	0	16.0	××	610	
Butter, garlic, 1 tbsp, 20g	0	16.0	××	610	
Butter, reduced fat, 1 tbsp, 20g	0	8.0	××	320	
Butter/oil spread, 1 tbsp, 20g	0	16.0	××	610	
Butter/oil spread, Devondale Extra Soft, 1 tbsp	0	12.0	××	435	
Butter/oil spread, Farmers Blend, 1 tbsp	0	12.0	××	435	
Butter/oil spread, reduced fat, 1 tbsp, 20g	0	10.0	××	380	
Buttermilk, 250 mL	0	5.0	×	575	✓
Buttermilk, low fat, 250 mL	0	1.5	×	330	✓
Buttermilk, skim, 250 mL	0	0		385	✓
Butterscotch sauce, 1/4 cup	0	16.0	××	965	××
Butterscotch, 25g	0	2.0	×	440	××
Cabbage rolls, Lebanese, 3 small, 250g	1.0	10.0	✓	1290	
Cabbage rolls, meat filling, each	7.0	9.0	×	800	
Cabbage, Chinese, 1/2 cup, 40g	1.0	0		30	
Cabbage, green, raw, 1/2 cup, 40g	0.5	0		25	
Cabbage, mustard, (gaai choi), 75g	1.5	0		50	
Cabbage, mustard, raw, 1/2 cup, 40g	1.0	0		25	
Cabbage, red, cooked, 1/2 cup, 60g	2.0	0		50	
Cabbage, red, raw, 1/2 cup, 40g	1.5	0		40	
Cabbage, Savoy, raw, 1/2 cup, 40g	1.5	0		30	
Cabbage, Savoy, steamed, 1/2 cup, 65g	2.0	0		45	
Cabbage, white, raw, 1/2 cup, 40g	1.5	0		30	

Food	Fibre g	Fat g	Fat Rating	Energy kJ	Carb Rating
Caesar salad with chicken, average serve	5.0	39.0	××	2800	
Caesar salad, average serve, 280g	4.5	30.0	××	1850	
Caesar salad, supermarket mix, 1 serve, 113g	1.0	2.5	✓	365	
Cake, angel, 1/10 20cm cake	0.5	0		760	××
Cake, apple, 1/6 18 cm cake	3.0	10.0	×	1060	××
Cake, Armenian nutmeg, 1/8 29 cm cake	5.0	22.0	××	1775	××
Cake, banana, 50g (small) slice, no icing	1.5	7.0	××	530	××
Cake, Black forest cherry, 1/10 average cake	2.0	34.0	××	2400	××
Cake, Black forest, purchased slice, 85g	0.5	16.5	××	1225	××
Cake, butter, 1/8 20 cm cake	1.5	15.0	××	1385	××
Cake, carrot, mad with oil, 1/12 average cake	3.0	42.0	✓	2740	××
Cake, cheesecake, baked, 1/8 of 20cm cake	1.5	55.0	××	3280	××
Cake, cheesecake, purchased, 100g slice	1.0	22.0	××	1420	××
Cake, chocolate eclairs, commercial, each	0.5	18.0	××	1110	××
Cake, chocolate eclairs, home-made, each	0.5	18.0	××	1235	××
Cake, chocolate purchased, 1/6 cake, 135g	5.0	35.5	××	2575	××
Cake, chocolate, plain, 1/12 average cake	0.5	12.0	××	1450	××
Cake, Christmas, 1 piece, 60g	1.5	6.5	××	815	×
Cake, cup, each	0.5	6.0	××	760	××
Cake, doughnut, custard-filled, 1, 90g	2.5	17.0	××	1350	××
Cake, doughnut, iced, 1, 80g	1.5	19.5	××	1425	××
Cake, doughnut, sugar, 1 50g	1.0	10.5	××	770	××
Cake, eclair, commercial, 1, 70g	0.5	18.0	××	1110	××
Cake, from mix, small slice, 50g	1.5	1.5	××	500	××
Cake, fruit, light, 1 piece, 75g	2.0	11.0	××	1075	×
Cake, fruit, rich, 1 piece, 75g	2.0	9.0	××	1375	×
Cake, hazelnut torte, 1/10 of cake	2.5	31.0	××	1690	××
Cake, lamington, commercial, 1, 75g	1.5	9.0	××	980	××
Cake, lamington, home-made, 1, 60g	1.0	6.0	××	815	××
Cake, Madeira, small slice, 60g	0.5	9.0	××	930	××
Cake, plain, iced, average slice, 60g	0.5	9.0	××	930	××

Food	Fibre g	Fat g	Fat Rating	Energy kJ	Carb Rating
Cake, plain, no icing, 50 g	0.5	8.0	××	740	××
Cake, rum baba, individual	1.5	8.5	××	1370	××
Cake, scone, home made, 1, 45g	1.0	6.5	×	685	✓
Cake, scone, home-made, wholemeal, 1, 50g	2.5	7.0	×	685	✓
Cake, sponge, home-made Genoise, 1/10	0.5	7.0	××	680	××
Cake, sponge, jam filled, 1 slice, 45g	0.5	2.0	×	575	××
Cake, sponge, vanilla, bought, 1/8 cake, 50g	0.5	7.0	××	675	××
Cake, sponge, Victoria, 1/10 cake	1.0	23.0	××	1670	××
Cake, Swiss roll, 1 slice, 35g	0.5	2.5	××	480	××
Cake, teacake, yeasted, 1 piece, 40g	1.5	3.0	×	500	✓
Cake, vanilla slice, commercial, 1, 135g	0.5	12.0	××	1150	××
Calamari rings, fried, 125g	0	12.0	✓	955	
Camp pie, canned, 60g	2.0	5.0	××	395	
Candle nuts, 1 tbsp, 20g	1.5	10.0	✓✓	485	
Cannellini beans, canned, 1 cup, 250g	16.0	1.5	✓	770	✓✓
Cannellini beans, dried, 100g	23.0	1.5	✓	1220	✓✓
Cannelloni, average serve	7.0	55.0	××	3900	✓
Canola oil, 1 tbsp	0	20.0	✓✓	740	
Cantaloupe 1 cup diced, 150g	1.5	0		135	
Cantaloupe, large wedge, 250g	2.5	0		230	
Capers, 1 tablespoon	0.5	0		10	
Capsicum, green, raw, 1/2 medium, 90g	1.5	0		60	
Capsicum, red, raw, 1/2 medium, 110g	1.5	0		115	
Capsicum, roasted, drained, 1/2 cup	1.5	1.5	✓	185	
Capsicum, yellow, raw, 1/2 medium, 100g	1.5	0		80	
Carambola (star fruit), 1 medium, 110g	2.0	0		255	✓
Caramel sauce, rich, average serve	0	35.0	××	1845	××
Caramel scroll (bun), 1, 120g	2.5	6.0	×	1535	×
Caramel syrup, 1/4 cup	0	0		820	××
Caramel Top'n'Fill, 1 can, 380g	0	27.0	××	4520	××
Caramel yumbats, each, 18g	0	4.5	××	360	××

Food	Fibre g	Fat g	Fat Rating	Energy kJ	Carb Rating
Caramels with nuts, 30g	1.0	5.0	×	540	××
Caramels, 4, 25g	0.5	3.0	××	420	××
Caramels, home-made, 1 piece, 28g	0	4.0	××	405	××
Caraway seeds, 1 tsp	1.0	1.0	✓	85	
Carbonara sauce, average serve, 150g	0	42.0	××	1930	
Carob bars, average, 45g bar	1.5	14.0	××	1015	××
Carob powder, 1 tbsp, 10g	0.5	0		155	✓
Carrot cake, 1/12 average cake	3.0	42.0	××	2740	××
Carrot juice, 1/2 cup, 125 mL	0	0		130	✓
Carrot, baby, 3, 50g	1.5	0		55	✓
Carrot, canned, 100g	3.0	0		85	✓
Carrot, cooked, 1/2 cup 70g	3.0	0		80	✓
Carrot, raw, 1 medium, 120g	4.0	0		100	✓
Casaba melon, 1 cup cubed, 160g	1.5	0		175	✓
Casaba melon, 1 slice, 150g	1.5	0		165	✓
Cashew nuts, raw, 50g	3.0	24.5	✓✓	1195	
Cashew nuts, roasted, 50g	3.0	25.5	✓✓	1310	
Cassava, cooked, 100g	2.0	0.5		550	✓
Cassoulet, average serve	10.5	50.0	××	3000	✓✓
Cauliflower, cooked, average serve, 100g	2.0	0		80	
Cauliflower, raw, 50g	1.0	0		40	
Caviar, 1 tsp	0	0		10	
Celeriac, cooked, 100g	5.0	0		130	
Celeriac, raw, 100g	4.5	0		120	
Celery, cooked, 1/2 cup, 75g	1.5	0		40	
Celery, raw, 1 stick 20cm long, 50g	1.0	0		25	
Cereal bar, Crunchy nut, 1, 33g	0.5	0.5		540	××
Cereal bar, Just Right, 1, 33g	2.0	1.0	✓	520	××
Cereal bar, Sustain, 1 33g	1.0	0.5		530	××
Cereal, 4 Brans, ½ cup, 50g	11.0	5.5	✓✓	820	✓✓
Cereal, All-Bran Fruit 'n Oats, 1/2 cup, 45g	9.0	2.0	✓	640	✓✓

Food	Fibre g	Fat g	Fat Rating	Energy kJ	Carb Rating
Cereal, All-bran, 3/4 cup, 45g	12.5	1.5	✓	630	✓✓
Cereal, Balance oat bran flakes, 1 cup, 30g	3.5	1.0	✓	480	✓
Cereal, barley bran, 20g	2.0	1.0	✓	270	✓✓
Cereal, Bart Simpson, No Problem O's, 1 cup, 45g	1.5	1.0		725	✗✗
Cereal, Bran Bix, 2 biscuits, 30g	6.5	1.0	✓	355	✓✓
Cereal, Bran Plus, 1/2 cup, 45g	20.5	2.0	✓	550	✓✓
Cereal, bran, processed, 1/2 cup, 45g	13.0	1.0	✓	495	✓
Cereal, branflakes, 1 cup, 40g	7.0	1.0	✓	570	✓✓
Cereal, Breakfast Blend, Bran, 25g	11.0	1.0	✓	335	✓✓
Cereal, Breakfast Blend, Lecithin, 25g	4.0	16.0	✓✓	675	✓
Cereal, Breakfast Blend, Nuts & Seeds, 25g	3.5	11.5	✓✓	585	✓✓
Cereal, Breakfast Blend, Tropical Fruit, 25g	1.0	0.5		385	✓
Cereal, Bush Foods, 1 cup, 30g	2.0	1.0	✓	460	✓
Cereal, Coco Bombs, 1 cup, 50g	1.0	1.5	✗	715	✗✗
Cereal, Coco pops, 1 cup, 45g	0	0.5		720	✗✗
Cereal, cornflakes, 1 cup, 30g	0	0.5		475	✗
Cereal, Crunchola, apple, 1/2 cup, 50g	6.0	3.0	✓✓	820	✓✓
Cereal, crunchy nut cornflakes, 1 cup, 45g	1.0	2.0	✓	750	✗
Cereal, Extra G, 1 cup, 35g	2.0	0		495	✓
Cereal, Fibre Plus, 1/2 cup, 45g	6.5	1.5	✓	630	✓✓
Cereal, Frosties, 1 cup, 40g	0.5	0		645	✗✗
Cereal, Fruit loops, 1 cup, 40g	0.5	0.5		655	✗✗
Cereal, Fruit 'n' bran flakes, 1 cup, 45g	6.0	1.0	✓	585	✓✓
Cereal, Fruit 'n' Nut Weeties, 1 cup, 45g	4.0	1.0	✓	620	✓
Cereal, Fruity bites, 1 cup, 35g	2.5	0.5		325	✓
Cereal, Fruity Bix, berry or apricot, 10	3.5	0.5		585	✓
Cereal, Good Start, 2 biscuits, 48g	4.5	2.5	✗	760	✓
Cereal, Gradual, honey toasted, ½ cup, 50g	3.0	3.5	✗	705	✓✓
Cereal, granola, 1/2 cup, 60g	2.5	1.5	✗	585	✓
Cereal, Granose, 2 biscuits, 30g	3.5	1.0	✓	400	✓

Food	Fibre g	Fat g	Fat Rating	Energy kJ	Carb Rating
Cereal, Guardian, 1 cup, 35g	6.5	0.5		420	✓✓
Cereal, Healthwise, bowel, 1 cup, 45g	9.5	1.5	✓	590	✓
Cereal, Healthwise, women, 1 cup, 45g	4.5	1.5	✓	640	✓
Cereal, Hi-Lite wholegrain, 40g	3.5	1.0	✓	505	✓✓
Cereal, Honey smacks, 1 cup, 40g	0.5	2.0	×	645	××
Cereal, Honey Weets, 1 cup, 30g	1.5	0		465	×
Cereal, instant porridge, 1 sachet	2.0	3.0	✓	520	✓
Cereal, Just Right, 1 cup, 45g	4.0	1.0	✓	670	✓
Cereal, Komplete muesli, 1/2 cup, 60g	4.5	5.5	×	975	✓
Cereal, Lite Bix, 2 biscuits, 30g	3.5	1.0	✓	400	✓
Cereal, Lite 'n' tasty, apricot, 1 cup, 45g	1.0	0		670	✓
Cereal, Lite Start Plus, 1 cup, 45g	2.0	0		720	✓
Cereal, LSA mix, 2 tbsp	4.5	8.5	✓✓	450	
Cereal, Milo, 1 cup, 30g	1.0	1.5	×	500	×
Cereal, Mini wheats, 15, 30g	3.0	0		435	✓
Cereal, muesli flakes, 1 cup, 40g	3.5	1.0	✓	560	✓
Cereal, muesli, Birchner, average serve, 230g	6.0	8.0	✓	1220	✓✓
Cereal, muesli, gluten free, 1 cup, 60g	2.5	2.0	✓	860	✓
Cereal, muesli, Lowans Natural, ½ cup, 50g	6.5	3.5	✓✓	715	✓✓
Cereal, muesli, natural, ½ cup, average, 60g	6.0	4.5	✓✓	835	✓✓
Cereal, muesli, Oven crisp, 50g	4.5	8.0	✓✓	890	✓✓
Cereal, muesli, Swiss natural, 60g	6.5	4.0	✓✓	910	✓✓
Cereal, muesli, toasted, average, 1/2 cup, 60g	5.5	8.5	×	1030	✓
Cereal, muesli, wheat free, yeast free, ½ cup, 40g	4.0	9.0	×	680	✓
Cereal, Multi-bran, 1/2 cup, 55g	11.5	7.0	✓✓	955	✓✓
Cereal, MultiFlakes, Soy & linseed, Fruit/nut, 1 cup, 45g	4.0	3.5	✓	685	✓
Cereal, MultiFlakes, Soy & linseed, Tropical, 1 cup, 45g	3.5	3.5	✓	630	✓✓
Cereal, Nut Feast, 1 cup, 45g	4.0	3.5	✓✓	750	✓
Cereal, Nutrigrain, 1 cup, 35g	1.0	0.5		560	×

Food	Fibre g	Fat g	Fat Rating	Energy kJ	Carb Rating
Cereal, Oat & Wheat Honeys, 1 cup, 50g	3.0	1.5	✓	675	××
Cereal, Oat bran bubbles, 1 cup, 30g	2.5	0		465	✓
Cereal, oat bran, crunchy, 1/2 cup, 50g	7.0	2.0	✓	720	✓
Cereal, oat bran, raw, 1/4 cup, 35g	6.0	3.0	✓	520	✓✓
Cereal, Oat Flakes, 1 cup, 50g	3.0	1.5	✓	765	✓
Cereal, Oat temptations, 1 sachet, 40g	3.0	2.5	✓✓	620	✓✓
Cereal, oats, high fibre, raw, 1/2 cup, 60g	8.0	5.5	✓✓	900	✓✓
Cereal, Oats, instant, brown sugar flavour, 1 sachet, 30g	2.5	2.0	✓✓	470	✓✓
Cereal, oats, rolled, 1/2 cup raw, 55g	4.0	4.5	✓✓	850	✓✓
Cereal, one minute oats, 1/2 cup, 45g	4.5	4.0	✓✓	690	✓
Cereal, OTS Fruity Bites, 1 cup, 35g	2.5	0.5		325	✓
Cereal, Puffed wheat, 1 cup, 30g	2.0	0.5		465	✓
Cereal, Ready Wheats, 20, 30g	3.0	1.0	✓	460	✓
Cereal, rice bran, crunchy 1 tbsp, 10g	2.5	2.0	✓	175	✓
Cereal, rice bran, crunchy, 1/2 cup, 55g	14.0	11.0	✓	975	✓
Cereal, rice bubbles, 1 cup, 30g	0.5	0		480	×
Cereal, Rice Crispies, 1 cup, 30g	0	0.5		460	×
Cereal, Rice Flakes with psyllium, 50g	4.0	1.0	✓	750	✓✓
Cereal, Ricies, 1 cup, 30g	0.5	0		465	✓
Cereal, San bran, 1/2 cup, 45g	15.0	4.0	✓	480	✓
Cereal, shredded wheat, 2 biscuits, 50g	6.5	0.5		665	✓
Cereal, Soy & linseed wheat bran, ¾ cup, 45g	13.5	0.5		705	✓✓
Cereal, Soy-tana, ¾ cup, 45g	9.0	0.5		705	✓✓
Cereal, Special K, 1 cup, 40g	1.0	0		630	✓
Cereal, Sportsplus, 1 cup, 45g	4.5	1.5	✓	680	✓
Cereal, sultana bran, 1 cup, 45g	6.5	1.0	✓	640	✓✓
Cereal, Sultanas and bran plus, 1 cup, 60g	7.5	1.5	✓	780	✓✓
Cereal, Sustain, 1 cup, 60g	4.5	1.5	✓	940	✓
Cereal, toasted muesli flakes, 1/2 cup, 45g	3.5	1.5	✓	645	✓
Cereal, Ultra rice with psyllium, 1 cup, 50g	1.5	0.5		780	✓

Food	Fibre g	Fat g	Fat Rating	Energy kJ	Carb Rating
Cereal, Vita Brits, 2 biscuits, 33g	4.0	0.5		500	✓
Cereal, Weeta Puffs, 1 cup, 20g	1.0	0.5		295	✓
Cereal, Weetbix Crunch, 1 cup, 35g	3.0	0.5		530	✓
Cereal, Weetbix Hi-Bran & soy, 2 biscuits, 40g	7.0	2.5	✓	520	✓
Cereal, Weetbix, 2 biscuits, 30g	3.5	0.5		420	✓
Cereal, Weetbix-Bix plus oatbran, 2 biscuits, 40g	5.5	1.5	✓	535	✓
Cereal, Weeties, 1 cup, 35g	4.5	1.0	✓	455	✓
Cereal, Weight Watchers fruit & fibre, 1/2 cup, 40g	5.0	1.0	✓	600	✓
Cereal, Weight Watchers muesli, 1/2 cup, 50g	6.0	1.0	✓	750	✓✓
Cereal, wheat bran, unprocessed, 2 tbsp, 12g	5.5	0.5		80	
Cereal, wheat flakes, 1 cup, 45g	5.5	1.0	✓	600	✓
Cereal, wheatgerm, 2 tbsp, 18g	3.5	1.5	✓✓	200	✓
Cereal,. Breakfast Blend, Seeds & Grains, 25g	6.5	3.0	✓✓	270	✓✓
Cereals, Crispex, cocoa, 1 cup, 30g	1.0	0.		475	×
Cereals, Crispex, honey, 1 cup, 30g	0.5	0		485	×
Champagne, 1 glass, 150 mL	0	0		405	
Champignon, canned, 1/2 cup, 100g	1.0	0.5		65	
Chapati wrap, 1, 44g	2.5	4.0	✓	520	✓
Chapati, home-made, 2 small	5.0	4.0	✓	665	✓
Chapati, Indian restaurant, average piece, 70g	4.5	1.5	✓	860	✓
Char sui barbecue sauce, 1 tbsp	0	0		45	
Chard, Swiss, 1/2 cup raw, 25g	0.5	0		20	
Chargrilled eggplant (deli), 100g	3.0	24.0	✓✓	1040	
Charlotte russe, average serve	0.5	21.0	××	1770	××
Cheese	0.5	22.0	×	1235	×
Cheese and bacon roll, 1, 100g	2.5	11.0	×	1230	✓
Cheese corn chips, 50g	5.0	14.0	××	1030	×
Cheese pastries, Greek, 1, 27g	0	6.0	×	310	×
Cheese sauce, made from packet, 1/2 cup	0	5.0	×	440	✓

Food	Fibre g	Fat g	Fat Rating	Energy kJ	Carb Rating
Cheese sauce, rich, for pasta, average serve, 150g	0	33.0	×	1630	✓
Cheese spread, 1 tbsp	0	6.0	×	290	
Cheese things, 50g	0.5	15.0	××	1065	××
Cheese tortellini, 100g	2.0	7.5	×	1285	✓
Cheese twist, snack, 12, 100g	0.5	14.5	××	1805	××
Cheese Twisties, 50g	0.5	14.0	××	1095	××
Cheese, bakers, 100g	0	2.5	×	390	
Cheese, blue brie, 30g	0	13.5	×	530	
Cheese, blue vein, 30g	0	10.0	×	480	
Cheese, brie, 30g	0	8.5	×	420	
Cheese, Caerphilly, 30g	0	9.5	×	465	
Cheese, camembert, 30g	0	8.0	×	390	
Cheese, cheddar slices, light singles,	0	3.5	×	215	
Cheese, cheddar, 30g	0	10.0	×	505	
Cheese, cheddar, low fat, Seven, 30g	0	2.0	×	240	
Cheese, cheddar, low fat, Super Light, 30g	0	3.0	×	295	
Cheese, cheddar, processed, 30g	0	8.0	×	415	
Cheese, cheddar, reduced fat, 30g	0	7.0	×	410	
Cheese, Cheshire, 30g	0	9.5	×	470	
Cheese, colby, 30g	0	10.0	×	480	
Cheese, cottage, 100g	0	9.5	×	610	
Cheese, cottage, low fat, 100g	0	1.0	×	375	
Cheese, cotto, 30g	0	3.5	×	265	
Cheese, cream, 30g	0	10.0	×	425	
Cheese, cream, light spreadable, 30g	0	4.0	×	210	
Cheese, creamed cottage, 100g	0	5.5	×	515	
Cheese, creamed cottage, low fat. 100g	0	2.5	×	410	
Cheese, double cream, 30g	0	12.0	××	560	
Cheese, double Gloucester, 30g	0	10.0	×	505	
Cheese, Edam, 30g	0	8.5	×	450	

Food	Fibre g	Fat g	Fat Rating	Energy kJ	Carb Rating
Cheese, farm, 30g	0	8.0	×	425	
Cheese, feta reduced fat, 30g	0	4.5	×	295	
Cheese, feta, 30g	0	7.5	×	380	
Cheese, feta, 97% fat free, 30g	0	1.0	×	190	
Cheese, fromage frais, fruit flavoured, 100g	0	4.0	×	455	
Cheese, fromage frais, low-fat, 100g	0	0	×	245	
Cheese, fromage frais, plain, 100g	0	7.0	×	470	
Cheese, fruit, 30g	0	7.0	×	405	
Cheese, Gloucester, 30g	0	10.5	×	510	
Cheese, goat, hard, 30g	0	11.0	×	565	
Cheese, goat, semi-soft, 30g	0	9.0	×	455	
Cheese, goat, soft, 30g	0	6.5	×	335	
Cheese, Gouda, 30g	0	9.0	×	465	
Cheese, Gruyere, 30g	0	10.0	×	510	
Cheese, haloumi, 30g	0	5.0	×	305	
Cheese, havarti, 30g	0	11.0	×	505	
Cheese, Jarlsberg Lite, 30g	0	5.0	×	340	
Cheese, Jarlsberg, 30g	0	9.0	×	475	
Cheese, Lancashire, 30g	0	9.5	×	465	
Cheese, Leicester, 30g	0	10.0	×	500	
Cheese, light cream, 30g	0	5.0	×	245	
Cheese, mascarpone, 30g	0	14.0	××	555	
Cheese, mozzarella, 30g	0	7.0	×	390	
Cheese, mozzarella, reduced fat, 30g	0	5.5	×	360	
Cheese, Neufchatel, 30g	0	8.5	×	380	
Cheese, Nimbin, 30g	0	10.0	×	500	
Cheese, Parmesan grated, 1 tbsp, 10g	0	3.0	×	180	
Cheese, Parmesan, 30g	0	10.0	×	565	
Cheese, pecorino, 30g	0	8.0	×	445	
Cheese, pepato, 30g	0	9.5	×	480	
Cheese, pizza, 1/2 cup grated, 60g	0	13.0	×	780	

Food	Fibre g	Fat g	Fat Rating	Energy kJ	Carb Rating
Cheese, Provolone, 30g	0	8.5	×	455	
Cheese, quark, 100 g	0	9.5	×	560	
Cheese, quark, low fat, 100g	0	1.0	×	320	
Cheese, raclette, 30g	0	9.0	×	460	
Cheese, ricotta smooth, Perfect, 100g	0	9.0	×	530	
Cheese, ricotta, 100g	0	11.5	×	615	
Cheese, ricotta, low fat, 100g	0	4.5	×	460	
Cheese, ricotta, reduced fat, 100g	0	8.5	×	555	
Cheese, ricotta, sheep's milk, 100g	0	11.0	×	635	
Cheese, Romano, 30g	0	8.5	×	470	
Cheese, samsoe, 30g	0	10.0	×	485	
Cheese, sheep's milk, Merino Fresh, 30g	0	6.5	×	380	
Cheese, soy, 30g	0	8.0	✓	390	
Cheese, Stilton, 30g	0	10.5	×	510	
Cheese, Swiss, 30g	0	9.0	×	475	
Cheese, Tilsit, 30g	0	9.0	×	465	
Cheese, Wensleydale, 30g	0	9.5	×	470	
Cheeseburger, 1	3.0	12.0	×	1220	✓
Cheesecake, baked, 1/8 of 20cm cake	1.5	55.0	××	3280	××
Cheesecake, individual, 1	1.0	7.0	××	735	××
Cheesecake, purchased, 100g slice	1.0	22.0	××	1420	××
Cheeseymite scroll, 1, 110g	3.0	11.5	×	1430	✓
Cheezels, 50g	0.5	13.5	××	1050	××
Cherimoya (custard apple), 100g	2.5	0		395	✓
Cherries canned in syrup, 1 cup, 250g	3.0	0		730	×
Cherries, canned, drained, 1 cup, 170g	3.0	0		500	✓
Cherries, fresh, weighed with stones, 100g	1.5	0		225	✓
Cherries, frozen, 100g	2.5	0		410	✓✓
Cherries, glace, 6, 30g	0.5	0		320	×
Cherry ripe bar, 85g	3.0	22.0	××	1710	××
Chestnuts, dried, 50g	6.0	2.5	✓✓	780	✓

Food	Fibre g	Fat g	Fat Rating	Energy kJ	Carb Rating
Chestnuts, fresh, 50g	3.0	1.5	✓✓	360	✓
Chewing gum, 10g	0	0		130	
Chick nuts (snack food), 50g	8.5	4.5	✓	800	✓✓
Chick pea flour (besan), 100g	13.5	5.5	✓✓	1330	✓
Chick peas, canned, drained, 1 cup, 180g	8.5	4.0	✓✓	735	✓✓
Chick peas, canned, Moroccan, 1 cup, 190g	18.0	1.5	✓✓	1100	✓✓
Chick peas, cooked, 1 cup, 160g	8.0	3.5	✓✓	820	✓✓
Chick peas, dried, ½ cup, 90g	12.0	5.0	✓✓	1220	✓✓
Chicken and almonds, average serve, 250g	2.0	24.5	✓	1440	
Chicken and sweet corn soup, 250 g bowl	4.0	3.0	✓	660	✓
Chicken breast, raw, no skin, 100g	0	2.5	✓	470	
Chicken curry, Vietnamese, average serve	5.5	20.0	✓	1330	
Chicken liver, fried, 120g	0	10.0	✓	810	
Chicken lovely legs (no skin), raw, 2	0	4.5	✓	620	
Chicken pastrami, 70g	0	2.0	×	395	
Chicken schnitzel, 1	1.0	10.0	×	1690	×
Chicken stock, ready made, 1 cup	0	0.5		95	
Chicken wing, raw, 4	0	19.0	×	1115	
Chicken wings, honey-soy, 1 serve, 250g	0	26.0	×	1840	
Chicken, biryani, average serve	5.0	60.0	×	3600	
Chicken, breast, baked, no skin, 100g	0	4.0	×	660	
Chicken, breast, baked, skin on, 100g	0	13.0	×	910	
Chicken, cacciatore, home-made, average serve	1.5	5.5	×	780	
Chicken, cacciatore, restaurant serve	1.5	31.0	×	1650	
Chicken, casserole/cream sauce, average serve	4.0	80.0	××	4000	
Chicken, chow mein, average serve, 250g	1.5	17.0	×	1060	
Chicken, coq au vin, ¼ chicken	1.5	28.0	×	1850	
Chicken, crispy skin, restaurant, 200g	0	21.0	×	1500	
Chicken, curry, Indian, average serve, 200g	2.0	32.0	×	1700	
Chicken, curry, Thai, coconut, average serve	1.5	22.0	×	1430	
Chicken, drumsticks, baked no skin, 2	0	9.0	✓	750	

Food	Fibre g	Fat g	Fat Rating	Energy kJ	Carb Rating
Chicken, drumsticks, baked. skin on, 2	0	14.0	✓	960	
Chicken, fillet burger, 1, 170g	1.0	22.5	×	1785	✓
Chicken, fried, take away, average piece	0	15.0	×	900	
Chicken, Kiev, home-made, average serve	2.5	54.0	×	3410	×
Chicken, lemon, Chinese, average serve	0	27.0	×	1770	
Chicken, liver pate, home-made, 100g	0	11.0	×	560	
Chicken, nuggets, 6	0	21.0	××	1560	×
Chicken, pieces, skin included, ¼ chicken	0	26.0	×	1600	
Chicken, Red Rooster, ¼ chicken, 240g	0	35.0	×	2460	
Chicken, Red Rooster, original, per piece	0	12.0	×	790	
Chicken, rissoles, 100g	0.5	13.5	××	900	×
Chicken, roast, supermarket, 250g	0	30.0	×	1860	×
Chicken, roll (sausage), 50g	0.5	4.5	×	330	×
Chicken, rotisserie, breast quarter, skin included	0	12.5	×	900	
Chicken, rotisserie, leg quarter, skin included	0	18.5	×	1120	
Chicken, smoked, 75g	0	7.5	✓	520	
Chicken, spicy skin free, centre breast, 115g	0	5.0	×	715	
Chicken, spicy skin free, drumstick, 75g	0	3.5	×	480	
Chicken, spicy skin free, side breast, 115g	0	3.0	×	460	
Chicken, spicy skin free, thigh, 120g	0	8.5	×	670	
Chicken, spicy skin free, wing, 75g	0	2.5	×	480	
Chicken, Tandoori, ¼ chicken	0.5	14.0	×	1400	
Chicken, Teriyaki, average serve	0	8.0	×	1160	
Chicken, thigh with skin and fat, 100g	0	15.0	×	1000	
Chicken, thigh, no skin, 100g	0	4.0	×	500	
Chicken, Tikka, average serve 275g	0	24.5	×	2120	
Chicory greens, raw, 1/2 cup, 80g	1.5	0		40	
Chiko roll, 1, 165g	2.0	17.0	××	1560	××
Chilli con carne, home-made, average serve	5.5	24.0	×	1650	✓✓
Chilli con carne, take-away, average serveg	8.0	21.0	××	1580	✓✓

Food	Fibre g	Fat g	Fat Rating	Energy kJ	Carb Rating
Chilli prawns, average serve	1.0	10.0	✓	620	
Chilli sauce, Asia at Home, ¼ cup	0	0		190	
Chilli sauce, stir-fry, 1 serve, 70g	0	0.5		530	×
Chilli sauce, sweet, 1 tbsp	0.5	1.5	✓	265	×
Chilli, banana, 1, 80g	1.0	0		45	
Chilli, long thin, 1, 80g	2.0	0		80	
Chilli, small green, 1, 20g	0.5	0		15	
Chilli, small red, 1, 20g	0.5	0		25	
Chinese cabbage, 2 cups	1.0	0		35	
Chinese chives, 1 tbsp	0	0		5	
Chinese flowering cabbage, 100g	3.0	0		50	
Chinese garland chrysanthemum, 100g	3.5	0		50	
Chinese mustard cabbage, 100g	2.0	0		60	
Chinese noodles, long life, 100g	3.0	0.5		1475	✓✓
Chinese spinach, 100g	4.5	0		70	
Chinese water spinach, 100g	3.0	0		90	
Chinese watercress, 100g	4.0	0		80	
Chinese white cabbage, 100g	2.5	0		45	
Chinese yard long beans, 100g	4.5	0		95	
Chips, see potato chips or crisps					
Chives, fresh, 2 tbsp	0	0		5	
Chocolate cake, plain, 1/12 average cake	0.5	12.0	××	1450	××
Chocolate cake, rich, 1/6 20 cm cake	3.0	43.0	××	3600	××
Chocolate creme eggs, small, each, 18g	0	3.0	××	290	××
Chocolate eclair, home-made, each	0.5	18.0	××	1235	××
Chocolate eclairs, commercial, each	0.5	18.0	××	1110	××
Chocolate fudge sauce, 1/4 cup	0	22.5	××	1530	××
Chocolate fudge, 50g	0	12.0	××	955	××
Chocolate hazelnut 'bread', ½ packet, 55g	0.5	4.5	✓	955	××
Chocolate hazelnut spread, 1 tbsp, 25g	0.5	8.5	×	575	××
Chocolate malted milkshake, 275 mL	0	12.0	×	1160	×

Food	Fibre g	Fat g	Fat Rating	Energy kJ	Carb Rating
Chocolate mousse, rich, average serve, 150 mL	0	27.0	××	2265	××
Chocolate mud cake, average slice	4.0	82.0	××	4670	××
Chocolate profiteroles, 1, 5cm x 75 cm	0.5	14.0	××	835	××
Chocolate pudding, steamed, average serve	2.0	15.0	××	1470	××
Chocolate sauce, home-made, 1/4 cup	0	6.0	××	650	××
Chocolate self-saucing pudding, average serve	1.5	10.0	××	1700	××
Chocolate shake, large, 420g	0	14.5	×	1940	×
Chocolate shake, regular, 300g	0	10.5	×	1410	×
Chocolate souffle, hot, home-made	0.5	13.0	××	1165	××
Chocolate souffle, restaurant, average serve	1.0	24.0	××	1925	××
Chocolate spread, 1 tbsp, 30g	0	9.0	××	665	××
Chocolate, dark, 50g block	0.5	14.0	××	1085	××
Chocolate, drinking, 18g + 200mL milk	0	8.5	×	870	××
Chocolate, drinking, 18g + 200mL skim milk	0	0.5		590	××
Chocolate, drinking, powder, 20g	0	1.0	×	310	××
Chocolate, fruit/nut, 6 squares, 30g	1.5	9.0	××	640	××
Chocolate, Lite, 75g bar	0	21.0	××	1250	××
Chocolate, milk, 10 squares, 50g	0.5	13.5	××	1080	××
Chocolate, milk, 100g block	1.0	27.5	××	2160	××
Chocolate, milk, filled, 100g	0	25.0	××	2010	××
Chocolate, milk, with nuts, 100g	5.0	30.0	××	2140	××
Chocolate, white, 50g	0	15.5	××	1105	××
Chocolate, yumbats, each square, 22.5g	0	6.0	××	485	××
Chocolates, cream filling, 2, 18g	0	4.5	××	360	××
Chocolates, with nut, 200g block	5.0	29.5	××	2140	××
Choko, (chayote), ½ medium, 85g	1.5	0		65	
Chorizo sausage, 100g	0	38.0	×	1900	
Chow mein, combination, average serve	5.0	25.0	×	2650	✓
Chow mein, prawn, average serve	0.5	33.0	×	1675	✓
Christmas cake, 1 piece, 60g	1.5	6.5	××	815	×
Christmas pudding, rich, 1/10 pudding	7.0	34.0	××	3640	×

Food	Fibre g	Fat g	Fat Rating	Energy kJ	Carb Rating
Chrysanthemum garland, 50g	1.0	0		25	
Chuck steak, see beef	0	0			
Chutney, fruit, 1 tbsp	0.5	0		145	×
Chutney, mango, home-made, 1 tbsp	0.5	0		125	×
Cider, alcoholic, 250 mL	0	0		400	
Cider, alcoholic, sweet, 250 mL	0	0		560	×
Cider, non alcoholic, 250 mL	0	0		415	×
Cinnamon scroll (bun), 1, 90g	3.0	3.0	✓	1100	✓
Cinnamon toast, 1 slice	1.0	7.0	×	600	✓
Clementines (mandarins), each	1.5	0		120	✓✓
Club sandwich, 1 (3 slices bread B.L T and cheese)	4.0	34.0	×	2440	✓
Club sandwich, bacon, lettuce, tomato, crisps	6.0	23.0	×	2000	✓
Cockles, 6, 30g	0	0		60	
Cocktails: Bloody Mary	0	0		520	
Cocktails: Brandy Alexander, 90 mL	0	15.0	××	1175	
Cocktails: Daiquiri	0	0		620	
Cocktails: Egg nog, 180 mL	0	18.5	××	1300	
Cocktails: Mimosa, 130 mL	0	0		420	
Cocktails: Singapore Sling, 150 mL	0	0		935	
Cocktails: Tequila Sunrise, 150 mL	0	0		650	
Cocktails: White Russian, 90 mL	0	13.0	××	1185	
Coco pops, see cereals					
Cocoa powder, 1 tbsp, 15g	0.5	2.0	×	190	
Coconut cream , fresh (grated coconut), 1 cup, 250mL	0	85.0	××	3615	
Coconut cream, block, 100 g	1.0	69.0	××	2760	
Coconut lime pie, average slice	3.0	50.0	××	3800	××
Coconut milk (cream), canned, 1 cup, 250mL	0	48.0	××	1860	
Coconut milk from centre of coconut, 1 cup	0	1.0	×	235	
Coconut milk, Lite, average, 1 cup, 250mL	0	12.5	××	650	
Coconut oil, 1 tbsp	0	20.0	××	740	

Food	Fibre g	Fat g	Fat Rating	Energy kJ	Carb Rating
Coconut, desiccated, 1 tbsp, 10g	1.5	6.5	××	260	
Coconut, fresh, 50g	4.0	14.5	××	560	
Coconut, health bar, 1, 45g	3.5	12.0	××	795	
Coconut, ice cream, Thai, 2 scoops	1.0	27.0	××	1220	×
Coconut, ice, 1 piece, 30g	1.5	9.0	××	615	××
Coconut, marshmallows, 1	0.5	0.5		225	××
Cod liver oil, 1 tbsp	0	20.0	✓	740	
Cod, smoked, cooked, 150g	0	2.0	✓✓	595	
Coffee & chicory essence, 1 tsp	0	0		45	
Coffee & date bun, 1, 85g	3.5	1.0	✓	985	✓
Coffee, cappuccino, latte or flat white, 160 mL	0	3.0	×	220	✓✓
Coffee, cappuccino, latte, flat white, skim, 160 mL	0	0		120	✓✓
Coffee, espresso, 100 mL	0	0		10	
Coffee, instant, 1 tspn	0	0		10	
Coffee, latte, mug	0	5.0	×	325	✓✓
Coffee, Vienna, 175 mL	0	17.0	××	780	✓
Coffee, with milk added, 250mL mug	0	1.0	×	65	
Coffee, with skim milk added, 250mL mug	0	0		40	
Coffeemate, 15mL	0	2.0	×	195	×
Cointreau, 1 glass, 40 mL	0	0		525	×
Cola soft drink, 1 can, 370 mL	0	0		650	××
Cola soft drink, 600 mL	0	0		1000	××
Coleslaw salad, lite, supermarket, 100g	2.5	2.0	✓	275	
Coleslaw salad, supermarket, 100g	2.5	10.0	✓	555	
Coleslaw, canned, 100g	3.0	6.0	✓	370	
Coleslaw, dressing, 2 tbsp	0	12.0	✓	530	
Coleslaw, dressing, reduced fat, 2 tbsp	0	1.0	✓	170	
Coleslaw, home-made, 1 cup, 150g	4.0	8.0	✓	500	
Coleslaw, take-away, 100g	2.5	4.0	✓	395	
Combination soup, average bowl	2.0	15.0	✓	775	✓

Food	Fibre g	Fat g	Fat Rating	Energy kJ	Carb Rating
Confectionery, chocolate honeycomb & nut bar, 1, 33g	0.5	5.0	××	615	××
Confectionery, LCM bars, average, 1	0	2.0	×	360	××
Confectionery, space food sticks, 1, 17g	0	3.0	×	300	×
Consomme, beef, 1 cup, 250 mL	0	0		135	
Cookies, McDonalds, 1	1.5	8.0	××	1170	××
Cooking oil, solid, 1 tbsp	0	20.0	××	740	
Copha, 100g	0	100.0	××	3700	
Coq au vin, average serve	1.5	28.0	×	1850	
Cordial, blackcurrant, diluted 1 in 5, 250 mL	0	0		430	××
Cordial, citrus, 25% juice, diluted 1 in 5, 250 mL	0	0		355	××
Cordial, citrus, 60% juice, diluted 1 in 5, 250 mL	0	0		395	××
Cordial, lime juice, diluted 1 in 5, 250 mL	0	0		365	××
Coriander, fresh, 1/2 cup chopped, 15g	0	0		15	
Coriander. Fresh, ¼ cup	0.5	0		10	
Corn chips, flavoured, 50g	5.0	14.5	××	1040	×
Corn chips, low fat, baked, 50g	5.0	1.5	✓	860	×
Corn chips, plain, 50g	5.0	13.5	××	990	×
Corn oil, 1 tbsp	0	20.0	✓	740	
Corn pasta, dry, 100g	11.0	2.0	✓	1495	✓
Corn, baby, canned, 6, 100g	3.5	0		75	✓
Corn, canned, 1 cup, 125g	4.0	1.5	✓	495	✓
Corn, creamed, canned, 1/2 cup, 125g	4.5	1.0	✓	425	✓
Corn, on the cob, 1 average, 150g	5.0	1.5	✓	440	✓✓
Cornbread, 140g slice	3.0	9.5	×	1240	✓
Corned beef & cereal, canned, 100g	1.5	13.5	×	825	✓
Corned beef, boiled, 100g, lean & fat	0	23.5	×	1300	
Corned beef, boiled, 100g, lean only	0	10.0	×	890	
Corned beef, canned, 100g	0	11.0	×	805	
Corned silverside, cold, 60g	0	1.5	×	250	

Food	Fibre g	Fat g	Fat Rating	Energy kJ	Carb Rating
Cornflakes, see cereal					
Cornflour, 1 tbsp, 10g	0	0		155	✓
Cornish pastie,1, 175g	2.0	35.5	××	2430	✓
Cornmeal, 100g	4.5	3.5	✓	1475	✓✓
Cottonseed oil, hydrogenated, 20g	0	20.0	××	740	
Courgettes, 100g	1.5	0		75	
Couscous, dry, ½ cup, 90g	2.0	1.0	✓	855	✓
Crab in black bean sauce, average serve, 150g	3.0	15.0	✓	965	
Crab sticks, 100g	0	0.5		290	
Crab, blue swimmer, 100g	0	1.0	✓✓	365	
Crab, canned, 100g	0	0.5		225	
Crab, spanner, 100g	0	1.0	✓	360	
Crabapples, 1 medium or 2 small, 60g	n/a	0		190	✓
Crackers, cheese, 4 small, 16g	0.5	4.0	××	315	××
Crackers, chicken flavoured, 8 small, 20g	0.5	5.0	××	410	××
Crackers, flaky texture, 6 small, 24g	0.5	4.0	××	415	×
Crackers, high fibre, 4, 25g	2.0	4.0	××	450	×
Crackers, Jatz, 6, 25g	0.5	5.0	××	460	×
Crackers, Lites, wholemeal, 2 (12.5g)	1.0	0.5		195	✓
Crackers, Premium, 6, 22g	0.5	4.0	××	425	×
Crackers, rice, 10, 20g	0.5	0.5		85	×
Crackers, Saltines, 3, 22g	0.5	4.5	××	420	×
Crackers, Sao, 3, 27g	0.5	4.0	××	485	×
Crackers, Thin Captain, 4, 22g	0.5	1.5	××	375	×
Crackers, Vita Wheat, 4, 25g	3.0	2.5	✓	410	✓
Crackers, water, 2. 15g	1.0	2.0	×	280	×
Crackers, water, sesame, 4 (13g)	0.5	1.5	×	230	×
Crackers, wholemeal & sesame, 4, 22g	1.5	3.5	×	400	✓
Crackers, wholemeal, 6, 22g	2.0	3.0	×	385	✓
Crackling, snack foods, 25g	0	7.0	××	510	
Craisins, 50g	2.5	0		680	✓

Food	Fibre g	Fat g	Fat Rating	Energy kJ	Carb Rating
Cranberries, fresh, 100g	4.0	0		205	✓
Cranberry sauce, 1 tbsp	0	0		125	×
Crayfish, cooked, farmed, 100g	0	1.5	✓✓	365	
Crayfish, cooked, wild, 100g	0	1.0	✓✓	345	
Cream caramel, 1/2 cup	0	16.0	××	1270	××
Cream cheese, light, 50g	0	8.5	××	410	
Cream horn, 1 65g	0.5	23.5	××	1170	××
Cream puff, each	0	18.0	××	930	××
Cream, canned, pressure pack, 100 mL	0	5.0	××	230	
Cream, clotted, 2 tbsp	0	25.0	××	965	
Cream, Dairy Whip, 100mL	0	10.5	××	465	
Cream, double, 2 tbsp	0	19.0	××	740	
Cream, light, 18% fat, 2 tbsp	0	7.0	××	280	
Cream, regular or thickened, 35% fat, 2 tbsp	0	14.0	××	560	
Cream, regular, 35% fat, 1 cup, 250mL	0	89.0	××	3500	
Cream, rich, 48% fat, 2 tbsp	0	19.0	××	740	
Cream, sour lite, 2 tbsp	0	8.0	××	350	
Cream, sour, 1/2 cup. 125g	0	46.0	××	1850	
Cream, sour, 2 tbsp	0	16.0	××	625	
Cream, sour, extra lite, 2 tbsp	0	5.0	××	270	
Cream, whipped, average serve, 1/4 cup, 40g	0	14.0	××	560	
Creme Anglais, 1/2 cup	0	8.0	××	765	×
Creme brulee, small pot, made with cream	0	50.0	××	2180	××
Creme caramel (1/2 cream, 1/2 milk), average serve	0	33.0	××	1560	××
Crepe, commercial, 1, 40g	0	6.0	✓	550	✓
Crepe, homemade plain, 1, 18cm diameter	0.5	2.5	×	275	✓
Crepes suzette, 2 filled crepes	2.0	29.0	××	1925	××
Cress, 1/4 cup, 15g	0.5	0		20	
Crispbread, puffed rye, 4, 22g	3.0	0.5		295	✓
Crispbread, puffed wholemeal, 4, 22g	1.5	1.0	✓	340	✓

Food	Fibre g	Fat g	Fat Rating	Energy kJ	Carb Rating
Crispbread, puffed, 4, 22g	0.5	1.0	✓	360	✓
Crispbread, Ryvita, 2 slices	2.5	2.0	✓	340	✓
Crispbread, wholemeal, 4, 25g	3.0	2.5	✓	425	✓
Crisps, apple, 50g	n/a	12.5	××	980	×
Crisps, bagel, 50g	1.5	6.5	✓	910	×
Crisps, bakers, 50g	1.0	7.5	✓	955	✓
Crisps, chick pea, 50g	4.5	18.0	××	1130	✓
Crisps, corn, flavoured, 50g	5.0	14.5	××	1040	×
Crisps, corn, low fat, 50g	5.0	1.5	✓	860	×
Crisps, corn, plain, 50g	5.0	13.5	××	990	×
Crisps, Pharo, average, 50g	2.5	3.0	×	850	×
Crisps, pita, 50g	1.5	8.5	×	910	✓
Crisps, potato, 50g	6.0	16.0	××	1050	×
Crisps, potato, flavoured, 50g	6.0	16.5	××	1085	×
Crisps, potato, Lites, 50g	6.0	16.5	××	1065	×
Crisps, sour cream & chive, 50g	1.5	8.5	×	555	×
Crisps, soy, 50g	2.5	12.0	✓	1040	×
Crisps, tortilla, 50g	4.0	11.0	✓	970	✓
Crisps, vege, 50g	1.5	10.5	××	1035	×
Crocodile, 100g	0	1.0	✓	n/a	
Croissant, 1, 70g	2.0	16.5	××	1150	×
Croissant, Bakers delight, 1, 85g	2.5	11.0	××	1330	×
Croissant, Bakers delight, chocolate, 1, 85g	2.5	11.0	××	1330	×
Croissant, ham and cheese	2.0	24.5	××	1600	×
Croissant. mini, 17g	0.5	4.0	××	280	×
Crostoli, 3 biscuits, 24g	0	1.5	×	245	×
Croutons, herb & garlic, 40g	1.5	3.0	×	670	✓
Crumpet, 1, 50g	1.0	0		390	✓
Crumpet, wholemeal, 1, 50g	1.5	0.5		355	✓
Crunchola, apple, ½ cup, 50g	6.0	3.0	✓✓	820	✓✓
Crunchy nut cornflakes, see cereal					

Food	Fibre g	Fat g	Fat Rating	Energy kJ	Carb Rating
Cucumber, 6 slices, 45g	0.5	0		20	
Cucumber, apple, ¼ medium, 80g	1.0	0		25	
Cucumber, green, 1 average, unpeeled, 250g	3.0	0		100	
Cucumber, Lebanese, 1 average, 130g	1.5	0		65	
Cucumber, telegraph, ¼ average, unpeeled, 95g	1.0	0		45	
Cumquats. 3 medium, 60g	3.0	0		160	✓
Cup cakes, each	0.5	6.0	××	760	××
Curly endive, average serve, 60g	1.5	0		25	
Currants, dried, ½ cup, 65g	4.0	0		730	✓
Currants, fresh, 1 cup, 110g	1.5	0		260	✓
Curry paste, 2 tbsp	1.5	8.5	✓	390	
Curry paste, Asia at home, 2 tbsp	n/a	4.0	✓	210	
Curry paste, average, 1 tbsp	0.5	1.0	✓	100	
Curry paste, Lemak, 2 tbsp	1.0	0		160	
Curry paste, Sharwoods tandoori, 2 tbsp	n/a	6.0	✓	355	
Curry paste, Sharwoods, 2 tbsp	n/a	12.0	✓	585	
Curry paste, Tandoori, 2 tbsp	1.0	1.0	✓	190	
Curry powder, 1 tbsp, 10g	2.3	1.0	✓	100	
Curry puffs (meat filling), Thai, each, 85g	0.5	31.0	××	1480	×
Curry sauce, green Thai, 1 serve, 93g	1.0	6.0	✓	420	×
Curry sauce, green Thai, with coconut cream, 1 serve	1.0	32.0	××	1500	×
Curry sauce, Korma, 100g	1.0	6.0	✓	295	
Curry sauce, red Thai, 1 serve, 93g	1.0	6.5	✓	525	×
Curry sauce, red Thai, with coconut cream, 1 serve	1.0	32.5	××	1610	×
Curry sauce, Vindaloo with coconut milk, ¼ packet	0	25.0	××	1145	×
Curry sauce, Vindaloo, 1 serve, 93g	0.5	9.0	✓	520	
Curry, beef vindaloo, average serve	2.0	35.0	××	2030	
Curry, prawn & coconut, average serve	1.0	21.0	××	1290	
Custard apple, 100g	2.5	0		305	✓

Food	Fibre g	Fat g	Fat Rating	Energy kJ	Carb Rating
Custard pie, average serve	0.5	23.0	××	1690	××
Custard powder, 1 tbsp, 10g	0	0		150	
Custard sauce, 1/2 cup	0	5.0	×	435	✓
Custard scroll bun, 90g	2.0	7.0	×	1145	×
Custard tart, 1 average, 150g	1.5	24.0	××	1740	××
Custard, baked, average serve	0	11.0	×	930	×
Custard, bread & butter, average serve	1.5	18.0	××	1530	×
Custard, creme Anglais, ½ cup	0	8.0	×	765	×
Custard, egg, pouring, ½ cup	0	6.0	×	570	×
Custard, purchased, ½ cup	0	4.0	×	490	×
Custard, purchased, Lite, ½ cup	0	1.0	×	410	×
Custard, purchased, reduced fat, ½ cup	0	2.5	×	425	×
Cuttlefish, cooked, 100g	0	0.5		660	
Daiquiri	0	0		620	
Dairy blend spread, 1 tbsp	0	15.0	××	555	
Dairy blend reduced fat spread, 1 tbsp	0	9.0	××	340	
Dairy Whip, 100 mL	0	10.5	××	465	
Damper buns, commercial, 1, 75g	1.5	2.0	✓	820	✓
Damper, home-made, 1/6 20cm loaf	3.5	6.5	×	1580	✓
Dandelion greens, 1/2 cup	0.5	0		40	
Danish pastry, 1 small, 100g	2.5	15.5	××	1290	
Date, dried, 6, 50g	5.0	0.5		565	✓
Date, fresh, 2, 60g	2.0	0.5		320	✓
Deep-fried ice cream, average serve	2.0	35.0	××	2500	××
Dessert, apple charlotte, average serve	6.5	13.0	××	2150	××
Dessert, apple flan, French, 1/6 20 cm flan	4.5	18.5	××	1895	××
Dessert, apple pie, double crust, 1/6 pie	2.5	21.0	××	1515	××
Dessert, apple pie, frozen, 1/6 of pie, 135g	2.0	18.5	××	1365	××
Dessert, apple pie, home-made, 1/6 23 cm pie	5.5	28.0	××	2520	××
Dessert, apple strudel, home-made, 1/10 strudel	4.0	23.0	××	1800	××

Food	Fibre g	Fat g	Fat Rating	Energy kJ	Carb Rating
Dessert, apple strudel, puff pastry, average serve	4.0	34.0	××	2055	××
Dessert, banana split, average	4.0	32.0	×	2575	×
Dessert, blancmange, average serve	0	5.0	×	620	✓
Dessert, bombe Alaska, 1/6 average cake	1.0	21.0	××	1900	××
Dessert, bread & butter custard, average serve	1.5	18.0	××	1530	✓
Dessert, charlotte russe, average serve	0.5	21.0	××	1770	××
Dessert, chocolate mousse, average serve, 150 mL	0	27.0	××	2265	××
Dessert, chocolate pudding, steamed, average serve	2.0	15.0	××	1470	××
Dessert, chocolate self-saucing pudding, average serve	1.5	10.0	××	1700	××
Dessert, chocolate souffle, hot, home-made	0.5	13.0	××	1165	××
Dessert, coconut custard, 150g	0	20.0	××	1230	×
Dessert, creme Anglaise, home made,1/2 cup	0	8.0	×	765	✓
Dessert, creme brulee, small pot, made with cream	0	50.0	××	2180	×
Dessert, custard pie, average piece	0.5	23.0	××	1690	××
Dessert, custard sauce, 1/2 cup	0	5.0	×	435	×
Dessert, custard tart, commercial, 1, 150g	1.5	24.0	××	1740	××
Dessert, custard, baked, 1/2 cup	0	7.0	×	540	×
Dessert, custard, egg, home made,1/2 cup	0	8.0	×	765	✓
Dessert, custard, purchased, ½ cup	0	4.0	×	490	×
Dessert, custard, purchased, reduced fat, ½ cup	0	2.5	×	425	×
Dessert, Duo de Mousse, 75g	0	7.5	××	590	××
Dessert, Duo raspberry ripple, 110g	0	2.0	×	520	××
Dessert, gulab jamen, average serve,	0.5	9.0	×	675	××
Dessert, lemon delicious, average serve	0.5	11.0	××	995	××
Dessert, lemon meringue pie 1/6 23 cm pie	0.5	18.0	××	1850	××
Dessert, peach Melba, average serve,	11.0	7.0	×	1500	×
Dessert, pecan pie, 1/8 23cm pie	2.5	33.0	××	2175	××
Dessert, plum pudding, rich, 1/10 pudding	5.5	19.5	××	2560	××

Food	Fibre g	Fat g	Fat Rating	Energy kJ	Carb Rating
Dessert, rice crPme, Attiki, 100g	0	3.0	×	495	×
Dessert, rice pudding, canned, 150g	0.5	4.0	×	560	×
Dessert, Rolo milk chocolate, 100g	0	12.0	××	965	××
Dessert, self-saucing pudding, 90g	1.0	6.0	×	215	××
Dessert, sorbet, average serve, 150g	0	0		360	××
Dessert, sponge pudding, canned, 75g	2.0	8.5	×	900	××
Dessert, summer pudding with cream	9.5	26.0	××	1995	✓
Dessert, summer pudding, average serve	9.5	1.5	✓	1075	✓
Dessert, sweet dumplings, 1	1.0	6.5	×	720	××
Dessert, tapioca cream, average serve	1.5	14.0	×	1180	×
Dessert, trifle, commercial, 125g	0.5	11.5	××	865	××
Dessert, trifle, home-made, average serve	1.0	23.0	××	2130	××
Dessert, upside-down cake, 1/8 of cake	0.5	10.0	×	750	××
Devilled chicken spread, 2 teaspoons	0	1.5	×	80	
Devilled ham spread, 2 teaspoons	0	1.0	×	70	
Devilled salmon spread, 2 teaspoons	0	1.0	✓	75	
Devondale Extra Soft spread, 1 tbsp	0	12.0	××	435	
Devon sausage, 50g	0.5	9.0	××	490	
Dhal, home-made, 1/2 cup	8.5	1.0	✓	890	✓✓
Dhal, 1/2 cup	6.5	5.5	✓	640	✓✓
Dijon mustard, 2 tsp	0	1.0	✓	65	
Dijonnaise dressing, 1 tbsp	0	6.0	✓	265	
Dim sim, 1, 50g	0.5	4.5	×	465	×
Dim sim, mini, 17g	0	1.5	×	160	×
Dinner rolls, bake at home, 1 roll, 40g	1.0	1.0	×	450	✓
Dip & crackers, smoky bacon, 1, 25g	0	5.5	××	395	×
Dip, spring onion with crackers, 1, 55g	1.0	12.5	××	820	×
Dip, French onion, 1 tbsp, 20g	0	6.5	××	275	
Dolmades, 3 average	2.0	15.0	✓	790	✓
Doner kebab, 1	8.0	24.0	×	2500	✓
Doughnut, custard-filled, 1, 90g	2.5	17.0	××	1350	××

Food	Fibre g	Fat g	Fat Rating	Energy kJ	Carb Rating
Doughnut, iced, 1, 80g	1.5	19.5	××	1425	××
Doughnut, sugar, 1 50g	1.0	10.5	××	770	××
Dove milk bar, 48g	1.0	14.5	××	1060	××
Dressing, balsamic, Neil Perry, 1 tbsp	0	10.0	✓	480	
Dressing, coleslaw, 1 tbsp	0	6.0	✓	330	
Dressing, coleslaw, reduced fat, 1 tbsp	0	2.0	✓	120	
Dressing, French, 1 tbsp	0	5.0	✓✓	220	
Dressing, French, home-made, (2/3 oil), 1 tbsp	0	13.0	✓✓	495	
Dressing, French, reduced fat, 1 tbsp	0	0		15	
Dressing, Italian, 1 tbsp	0	6.5	✓✓	260	
Dressing, Italian, reduced fat, 1 tbsp	0	0		25	
Dressing, soy, Neil Perry, 1 tbsp	0	4.5	✓	240	
Dressing, thousand island, 1 tbsp	0	4.5	✓	220	
Dressing, thousand island, reduced fat, 1 tbsp	0	2.0	✓	140	
Dried fruit & nuts, 50g	4.0	14.0	✓✓	900	✓✓
Dried fruit bar with seeds, 1, 45g	3.5	8.5	✓	765	✓
Dried fruit, mixed, 1/2 cup, 75g	4.0	1.0	✓	725	✓✓
Dripping, 1 tbsp	0	20.0	××	740	
Duck egg, 1, 70g	0	9.5	×	545	
Duck, roasted, breast only, meat & skin, ½ breast	0	12.0	✓	885	
Duck, roasted, lean only, 100g	0	9.5	✓	790	
Duck, roasted, leg, meat & skin, 1 portion	0	10.5	✓	835	
Duck, roasted, meat, fat and skin, 100g	0	28.5	✓	1410	
Duck, steamed/mushrooms, average serve, 200g	3.0	21.5	✓	1180	
Duck, wild, meat & skin, 100g	0	15.0	✓	885	
Duck, wild, meat only, 100g	0	4.5	✓	515	
Dumplings, sweet, , 1	1.0	6.5	×	720	××
Easter bun, 1 regular, 90g	3.0	4.0	×	1080	✓
Easter bun, 1 small, 45g	1.5	2.0	✓	540	✓
Eclair, chocolate, home-made, each	0.5	18.0	××	1235	××

Food	Fibre g	Fat g	Fat Rating	Energy kJ	Carb Rating
Eclair, commercial, 1, 70g	0.5	18.0	××	1110	××
Eel, raw, 100g	0	11.5	✓	680	
Egg, 1, raw, boiled or poached	0	5.5	✓	285	
Egg flip, 200 mL	0	9.5	×	690	✓
Egg nog, 125 mL glass	0	5.0	×	595	✓
Egg white, 1	0	0		50	
Egg yolk, 1	0	5.5	✓	250	
Egg, duck, 1, 70g	0	9.5	×	545	
Egg, fried, 1	0	8.5	×	410	
Egg, goose, 1, 140g	0	19.0	×	1115	
Egg, turtle, 100g	0	12.5	×	945	
Eggplant dip (baba ghannouj), average serve	5.5	12.0	✓✓	610	
Eggplant, baby, 4, 65g	1.5	0		50	
Eggplant, chargrilled (deli), 100g	3.0	24.0	✓✓	1040	
Eggplant, fried in a little oil, 100g	2.5	8.0	✓✓	375	
Eggplant, fried in oil, 100g	2.5	25.0	✓✓	1000	
Eggplant, grilled, 3 slices, 90g	2.5	0		65	
Eggplant, marinated in oil, 100g	2.5	25.0	✓✓	1000	
Eggplant, raw, 100g	2.5	0		70	
Eggs, Benedict, average serve, 2 eggs	1.5	52.0	×	2900	
Eggs, fried, 2, plus fried bacon	0	32.0	×	1660	
Eggs, omelette, plain or herbs, 2 eggs	0	18.0	×	860	
Eggs, poached, 2, plus lean grilled bacon	0	14.5	×	1010	
Eggs, scrambled, 2	0	18.0	×	860	
Elderberries, 1 cup, 140g	10.0	0		425	✓
Enchilada wrap, 1, 28g	1.0	2.5	×	365	✓
Enchilada, cheese and beef, 1, 190g	15.0	17.5	×	1350	✓
Enchilada, cheese, 1, 160g	15.0	19.0	×	1335	✓
Endive, Belgian, 1 head, 60g	1.0	0		30	
Endive, curly, 1/2 cup, 40g	1.0	0		20	
English muffin, 1	1.5	1.0	✓	575	✓

Food	Fibre g	Fat g	Fat Rating	Energy kJ	Carb Rating
Extra G, 1 cup, 35g	2.0	0		495	✓
Fajita wrap, 1, 25g	1.0	2.5	×	340	✓
Farmers Blend spread, 1 tbsp	0	12.0	××	435	
Feijoa, 1 large 50g	1.5	0		75	✓
Felafel, home-made, 2	3.0	9.5	✓	525	✓✓
Felafel, take-away, 2 small, each 30g	3.0	9.0	✓	595	✓✓
Fennel, 1/4 bulb steamed, 75g	3.0	0		65	
Fennel, raw, 1/2 cup sliced, 60g	2.0	0		45	
Feta, see under cheeses					
Fettuccine, fresh, 100g	3.0	1.5	×	1100	✓✓
Fibre Plus bars, average, 1, 37g	2.0	2.0	✓	550	×
Fibre Plus, 1/2 cup, 45g	6.5	1.5	✓	630	✓✓
Figs, dried, 3, 40g	5.5	0		385	✓
Figs, fresh raw, each, 60g	1.5	0		100	✓
Figs, glace, 100g	2.5	0		1035	×
Figs, semi-dried, sweetened, 3, 70g	8.0	0		325	✓
Fillet steak, grilled, trimmed, 1 small, 100g	0	10.0	×	880	
Filo pastry, 2 sheets, 34g	0.5	1.0	✓	440	✓
Finger bun, iced, 1, 85g	2.0	3.0	✓	1130	×
Finger bun, no icing, 1, 65g	2.0	3.0	✓	810	✓
Fish and chips, average serve	5.0	35.0	×	3000	✓
Fish balls, Asian, steamed, 2, 50g	0	2.5	✓✓	160	
Fish cakes, frozen, fried, medium, each, 80g	1.0	8.5	×	780	
Fish cakes, frozen, fried, small, each, 50g	0.5	6.5	×	485	
Fish cakes, large, each, 165g	3.5	24.0	×	1500	
Fish fingers, fried, 4, 110g	0.5	19.0	✓	1260	×
Fish fingers, grilled, 4, 100g	0.5	9.0	✓	890	×
Fish kedgeree, average serve, 200g	0.5	16.0	✓	1400	✓
Fish paste, 1 teaspoon	0	0.5		35	
Fish roe, black 10g	0	0.5		40	
Fish roe, red 10g	0	1.0	✓	65	

Food	Fibre g	Fat g	Fat Rating	Energy kJ	Carb Rating
Fish sauce, 1 tbsp	0	0		30	
Fish sauce, Vietnamese, 1 tbsp	0	1.0	✓	100	
Fish stick, crab-flavoured, 3, 105g	0	1.0	✓	400	
Fish, angel shark, grilled, 150g	0	0.5	✓✓	620	
Fish, Atlantic salmon, fresh, grilled, 150g	0	4.0	✓✓	765	
Fish, Australian salmon, grilled, 150g	0	1.5	✓✓	640	
Fish, average, grilled, 150g	0	1.0	✓✓	600	
Fish, barramundi, grilled, 150g	0	1.5	✓✓	620	
Fish, battered, 1 piece, 150g	0.5	23.5	✗	1590	
Fish, blackfish, grilled, 150g	0	1.0	✓✓	600	
Fish, blue eye cod, grilled, 150g	0	2.0	✓✓	640	
Fish, bream, grilled, 150g	0	1.0	✓✓	600	
Fish, canned, Australian salmon, 100g	0	1.0	✓✓	400	
Fish, canned, herring, 100g can, drained wt 70g	0	14.0	✓✓	610	
Fish, canned, herrings in tomato sauce, 100g	0	10.5	✓✓	735	
Fish, canned, pilchards in tomato sauce, 100g	0	5.5	✓✓	530	
Fish, canned, pink salmon, 100g, drained, 88g	0	6.0	✓✓	545	
Fish, canned, red salmon, 100g, drained, 88g	0	10.5	✓✓	720	
Fish, canned, sardines, in oil, 100g, drained, 80g	0	12.5	✓✓	760	
Fish, canned, sardines, in tomato sauce, 100g	0	11.5	✓✓	740	
Fish, canned, tuna, brine/water, 100g, drained, 80g	0	2.0	✓✓	415	
Fish, canned, tuna, in oil, 100g can, drained, 80g	0	11.0	✓✓	715	
Fish, canned, tuna, sandwich, canned in oil, 100g	0	8.0	✓✓	780	
Fish, chowder, average bowl	3.0	10.0	✓	850	
Fish, cocktail pieces, deep fried, 4, 120g	1.0	20.0	✗	1400	✗
Fish, crumbed, oven-cooked, 2 pieces, 140g	1.0	20.0	✗	1355	✗
Fish, crumbed, oven-fried, Lite, 2 pieces, 125g	2.5	8.5	✗	850	✗
Fish, fillet floured and fried in oil,	0	11.0	✓	400	

Food	Fibre g	Fat g	Fat Rating	Energy kJ	Carb Rating
Fish, fillet fried in solid oil or fat,	0	8.0	×	300	
Fish, fillet fried in unsaturated oil,	0	6.0	✓	220	
Fish, flathead, grilled, 150g	0	1.0	✓✓	570	
Fish, gemfish, grilled, 150g	0	4.0	✓✓	700	
Fish, jewfish, grilled, 150g	0	1.0	✓✓	540	
Fish, John dory, grilled, 150g	0	1.0	✓✓	570	
Fish, kingfish, grilled, 150g	0	1.0	✓✓	585	
Fish, kipper, baked, 100g	0	6.0	✓✓	465	
Fish, leather jacket, steamed, 150g	0	0.5	✓✓	525	
Fish, lemon sole, grilled, 150g	0	2.0	✓✓	515	
Fish, ling, grilled, 150g	0	0.5	✓✓	590	
Fish, mackerel, blue, grilled, 150g	0	5.5	✓✓	740	
Fish, mackerel, school, 150g	0	1.5	✓✓	590	
Fish, mackerel, Spanish, grilled, 150g	0	4.5	✓✓	700	
Fish, mirror dory, grilled, 150g	0	1.0	✓✓	435	
Fish, morwong, grilled, 150g	0	1.0	✓✓	590	
Fish, mullet, grilled, 150g	0	1.5	✓✓	615	
Fish, ocean perch, grilled, 150g	0	1.0	✓✓	600	
Fish, orange roughy, grilled, 150g	0	7.5	✓✓	830	
Fish, oreo, smooth, grilled, 150g	0	4.5	✓✓	760	
Fish, oreo, spiky, grilled, 150g	0	2.5	✓✓	670	
Fish, pan-fried, average serve, 200g	0	6.0	✓✓	1060	
Fish, pilchards, floured & fried, 120g	0	10.0	✓	740	
Fish, redfish, grilled, 150g	0	1.0	✓✓	600	
Fish, sea bream, grilled, 150g	0	1.5	✓✓	480	
Fish, sea perch, grilled, 150g	0	0.5	✓✓	480	
Fish, shark or flake, grilled, 150g	0	1.0	✓✓	610	
Fish, silver warehou, grilled, 150g	0	2.0	✓✓	650	
Fish, smoked cod, 150g	0	2.0	✓✓	595	
Fish, snapper, grilled, 150g	0	1.0	✓✓	590	
Fish, steamed, average, 1 piece, 150g	0	1.5	✓✓	600	

Food	Fibre g	Fat g	Fat Rating	Energy kJ	Carb Rating
Fish, swordfish, grilled, 150g	0	11.5	✓✓	845	
Fish, teraglin, grilled, 150g	0	1.5	✓✓	590	
Fish, trevally, grilled, 150g	0	2.0	✓✓	675	
Fish, trout, whole, baked, 1	0	3.0	✓✓	660	
Fish, tuna, fresh, grilled, 150g	0	1.0	✓✓	610	
Fish, whitebait, fried, 60g	0	28.5	×	1305	
Fish, whiting, King George, grilled, 150g	0	1.0	✓✓	580	
Fish, whiting, sand, grilled, 150g	0	1.0	✓✓	580	
Fish, wrasse, grilled, 150g	0	5.5	✓✓	785	
Fish, yellowfin tuna, grilled, 150g	0	1.0	✓✓	610	
Flake, grilled, 150g	0	1.0	✓✓	610	
Flaky pastry, average portion, 65g	1.0	26.0	××	1515	×
Flapjacks, 1, 15cm diameter	1.0	7.0	×	675	✓
Flathead, grilled, 150g	0	1.0	✓✓	570	
Flavoured milk, reduced fat, chocolate, 300 mL	0	5.0	×	760	✓
Flavoured milk, reduced fat, strawberry, 300 mL	0	4.5	×	775	✓
Flavoured, milk, chocolate, 300 mL	0	11.0	×	995	✓
Flavoured, milk, strawberry, 300 mL	0	10.5	×	975	✓
Florentines, 1, 40g	0.5	13.5	××	860	××
Flour, millet, 1 cup, 125g	13.0	2.5	✓	1410	✓✓
Flour, plain white, 1 cup, 140g	5.0	1.5	✓	2060	✓
Flour, rice, 1 tbsp, 12g	0	0		180	✓
Flour, rye, 1 cup, 140g	17.0	3.0	✓	1720	✓
Flour, self-raising, 1 cup, 140g	5.0	1.5	✓	1975	✓
Flour, wholemeal, 1 cup, 125g	17.0	3.0	✓	1755	✓✓
Flyte bar, 1, 40g	1.0	6.5	××	680	××
Focaccia, average piece, no filling, 100g	2.5	9.0	✓	1040	✓
Focaccia, baked supreme, ½, 170g	4.5	10.0	×	1370	✓
Focaccia, baked, bacon supreme, 1 piece, 180g	4.5	14.5	×	1900	×
Focaccia, baked, capsicum & mushroom, 1 piece, 160g	4.5	11.5	×	1680	✓

Food	Fibre g	Fat g	Fat Rating	Energy kJ	Carb Rating
Focaccia/avocado, bacon, cheese	5.0	60.0	×	3700	✓
Focaccia/eggplant, pesto, sun dried tomato, cheese	5.0	45.0	×	2700	✓
Focaccia/goats cheese, sun dried tomato, rocket	5.0	36.0	×	2275	✓
Fondue, including bread, average serve	2.5	31.0	×	2700	✓
Foule moudamass (broad beans), average, 280g	11.0	7.5	✓	855	✓✓
Frankfurt, cooked, 1 large or 4 cocktail, 105g	1.0	21.0	×	1090	
Frankfurt, slim, 1, 63g	1.0	5.5	×	345	
Freekah, 100g dry	16.5	3.0	✓	1470	✓✓
Freekah, cooked, 1 cup	9.0	1.5	✓	810	✓✓
French apple flan, 1/6 20 cm flan	4.5	18.5	××	1895	××
French crepe, commercial, 1, 40g	0	6.0	✓	550	✓
French dressing, 1 tbsp	0	5.0	✓✓	220	
French dressing, home-made, (2/3 oil), 1 tbsp	0	13.0	✓✓	495	
French dressing, reduced fat, 1 tbsp	0	0		15	
French fries, average serve	4.0	22.0	××	1700	✓
French fries, large	6.0	26.0	××	1790	✓
French onion dip, 1 tbsp, 20g	0.5	6.5	××	275	
French onion soup with cheese, average bowl	4.0	25.0	×	1800	✓
French onion soup, home-made, 1 bowl, 350g	1.5	7.5	×	445	✓
French toast, 1 slice	1.0	12.0	×	800	✓
Fresh cheese, Indian, 50g	0	11.0	×	780	
Fried rice, average plate (restaurant),	2.0	13.5	×	1490	✓
Fried rice, home-made, 1 cup, 160g	2.0	5.0	✓	885	✓
Frittata, average serve, 1/4 pie, 330g	5.0	12.0	×	920	
Fritters, banana, each	3.0	29.0	×	1840	✓
Fritto misto di mare (fried seafood), average serve	1.0	29.0	✓	2450	
Fromage blanc, 100g	0	6.5	×	405	
Fromage blanc, home-made, 1/4 cup	0	3.5	×	265	
Fromage frais, Danais, with fruit, average, 150g	0	5.5	×	775	✓

Food	Fibre g	Fat g	Fat Rating	Energy kJ	Carb Rating
Fromage frais, Frubelle, strawberry, 100g	0	5.0	×	590	✓
Fromage frais, Fruche, Light, 125g	0	0.5		460	✓
Fromage frais, Fruche, vanilla, 200g	0	8.0	×	970	✓
Fromage frais, Fruche, with fruit, average, 200g	0	6.0	×	955	✓
Fromage frais, low-fat, 100g	0	0	×	245	✓
Fromage frais, Petit Miam, 60g carton	0	4.0	×	350	✓
Fromage frais, plain, 100g	0	7.0	×	470	✓
Frosties, 1 cup, 40g	1.5	0.5		710	××
Frosty fruit iceblock, 1, 75mL	0	0		325	××
Frozen fruit 'n' yoghurt, 100g	0.5	5.0	×	590	✓
Frozen tea infusion, 1 cup	0	0		875	
Frozen yoghurt, Alfresko, 1, 180 mL	0	4.0	×	595	✓
Frozen yoghurt, apricot, 85g	0	4.5	×	535	✓
Frozen yoghurt, Baskin Robbins, low fat, 100g	0	3.0	×	480	✓
Frozen yoghurt, Baskin Robbins, non-fat, 100g	0	0		335	✓
Frozen yoghurt, Honey Hill Farms, non fat, 1 cone	0	1.0	×	460	✓
Frozen yoghurt, Honey Hill, reduced fat, 1 cone	0	0		380	✓
Frozen yoghurt, no fat, no sugar, 1 cone	0	0		190	✓
Frozen yoghurt, NZ natural, 180g	0	3.5	×	1075	✓
Frozen yoghurt, soft serve, Colombo, 100 mL	0	0.5		375	✓
Frozen yoghurt, soft serve, low fat, average	0	3.0	×	435	✓
Frozen yoghurt, soft serve, non fat, average	0	0		335	✓
Frozen yoghurt, strawberry, 85g	0	4.0	×	535	✓
Frozen, fruit yoghurt on stick, 70g	0	2.0	×	375	×
Fruccio, vanilla, 100 mL	0	1.5	×	315	×
Fruche, fruit flavoured, 200g	0	5.0	×	980	✓
Fruche, fruit flavoured, lite, 125g	0	0.5		460	✓
Fruche, lemon meringue, lite, 200g	0	1.0	×	640	✓
Fruche, on fruit, 200g	0	1.0	×	755	✓
Fruche, vanilla, 200g	0	8.0	×	910	✓

Food	Fibre g	Fat g	Fat Rating	Energy kJ	Carb Rating
Fruche, vanilla, lite, 200g	0	1.0	×	670	✓
Fruit bar, Aussie fruit slice, 1, 20g	n/a	0		125	✓
Fruit bars, IXL, average, 1, 20g	0	1.0	✓	315	××
Fruit bun loaf, 1 slice, 50g	1.5	2.0	✓	570	✓
Fruit bun, mini, 1 35g	1.0	1.0	✓	450	✓✓
Fruit cake, light, 1 piece, 75g	1.5	11.0	××	1080	×
Fruit cake, rich, 1 piece, 75g	2.0	8.5	××	1375	×
Fruit cocktail, canned in syrup, 1 cup	3.0	0		830	✓
Fruit fingers, each, 20g	1.5	2.0	×	320	×
Fruit gums, 6, 25g	0	0		185	××
Fruit juices, see juice					
Fruit loaf, 1 slice, 40g	1.0	2.0	×	515	✓
Fruit loops, 1 cup, 40g	0.5	0.5		655	××
Fruit mince pie, individual, 1	1.5	14.0	××	1185	××
Fruit 'n' bran flakes, 1 cup, 45g	6.0	1.0	✓	585	✓✓
Fruit roll-ups, average, 1, 15g	0	0.5		240	××
Fruit salad, canned in heavy syrup, 1 cup	3.0	0		830	×
Fruit salad, canned in syrup, drained, 1 cup	3.5	0		530	✓
Fruit salad, canned in water, 1 cup	3.5	0		310	✓
Fruit salad, fresh, average serve, 200g	3.5	0		475	✓
Fruit spread, 1 tbsp	0.5	0		140	×
Fruit straps, average, 1, 20g	0	0.5		215	××
Fruit twist bars, 1, 38g	1.5	1.0	×	540	××
Fruit, see individual entries					
Fruity Bix, berry or apricot, 10	3.5	0.5		585	✓
Fu juk (dried tofu), 100g	1.0	16.0	✓	1620	
Fudge brownies, 1 small, 40g	0.5	12.0	××	770	××
Fudge sundae, 1	0	10.5	××	1320	××
Fudge, chocolate, 50g	0	12.0	××	955	××
Fudge, vanilla, 50g	0	5.5	××	835	××
Gado gado, with peanut sauce	7.0	50.0	✓	2200	

Food	Fibre g	Fat g	Fat Rating	Energy kJ	Carb Rating
Gaii choi (mustard cabbage), 75g	1.5	0		50	
Galactbureko, Greek pastry, 1, 150g	1.0	13.0	✗✗	1345	✗
Galiko basil pesto, 1 tbsp	0.5	4.5	✓	210	
Garam masala powder, 1 tbsp	n/a	1.5	✓	160	
Garlic bread, ¼ French stick, 90g	2.0	27.0	✗✗	1550	✓
Garlic bread, fast food outlet, 1 roll, 156g	5.0	14.5	✗✗	2000	✓
Garlic powder, 1 tsp	0.5	0		25	
Garlic prawns, average serve, 150g	0	11.0	✓✓	765	
Garlic puree, 1 teaspoon	0	1.5	✓	80	
Garlic sausage, 50g	1.0	9.5	✗✗	515	
Garlic, 2 cloves, 6g	1.0	0		25	
Garlic, whole bulb, roasted, 50g	10.0	1.5	✓	215	
Gazpacho, large bowl	3.5	10.0	✓✓	930	✓
Gelati, chocolate, 100g serve	0	7.0	✗	700	✗
Gelati, hazelnut, 100g serve	0	6.5	✗	805	✗
Gelati, lemon sorbet, 100g serve	0	0.5		480	✗
Gelati, mango, 100g serve	0	1.5	✗	485	✗
Gelatine, 1 tbsp, 7.5g	0	0		110	
Gelato (non-dairy), 100g	0	0		660	✗
Gelato, vanilla, 100g	0	6.0	✗	700	✗
Gemfish, grilled, 150g	0	4.0	✓✓	700	
Ghee, 1 tbsp, 20g	0	20.0	✗✗	740	
Gherkins, pickled, each, 25g	0.5	0		15	
Gin, 1 nip, 30 mL	0	0		270	
Ginger ale, 1 glass, 250 mL	0	0		295	✗✗
Ginger, Buderim, 1 tbsp	0.5	0		245	✗
Ginger, ground, dried, 1 tsp	n/a	0		30	
Ginger, raw, sliced, 1 teaspoon	0	0		5	
Gingerbread, home-made, average slice, 80g	0.5	6.0	✗✗	980	✗✗
Glace cherries, 6, 30g	0.5	0		320	✗
Globe artichoke, 1 medium, 320g as purchased	1.5	0		105	

Food	Fibre g	Fat g	Fat Rating	Energy kJ	Carb Rating
Glucose powder, 1 tbsp	0	0		365	××
Glucose, liquid, 1 tbsp	0	0		255	××
Gluten-free bread, 30g slice	2.0	2.0	✓	290	✓
Gluten-free Chocolate Blitz biscuit, 1	1.5	3.5	×	350	××
Gluten-free Strawberry slice, 1, 50g	3.0	1.5	×	630	××
Gnocchi, fresh, uncooked, 100g	2.0	2.0	✓	975	✓
Gnocchi, Golden pasta, 200g	4.0	2.0	✓	1310	✓
Gnocchi, Golden pasta, pumpkin, 200g	2.0	1.0	✓	1740	✓
Gnocchi, potato, average serve	6.5	3.5	✓	2045	✓
Gnocchi, ready to cook, 100g	2.0	2.0	✓	960	✓
Gnocchi, semolina, with Parmesan, 300g	0.5	29.0	×	1590	✓
Goat cheese, see cheese					
Golden syrup dumplings, 1	1.0	6.5	××	720	××
Golden syrup, 1 tbsp, 25g	0	0		300	××
Good Start, 2 biscuits, 48g	4.5	2.5	×	760	✓
Goose egg, 1, 140g	0	19.0	×	1115	
Goose, roast, lean only, 100g	0	12.5	×	995	
Gooseberries, canned, 1 cup	6.0	0		775	✓
Gooseberries, fresh, 100g	3.0	0		230	✓
Gourd, bottle, 75g	2.0	0		40	
Gourd, ridge, 75g	1.5	0		55	
Gourd, wax, 75g	1.0	0		15	
Granola, 1/2 cup, 60g	2.5	1.5	×	585	✓
Grape juice, sweetened, 250 mL	0	0		640	✓
Grape juice, unsweetened, 250 mL	0	0		490	✓
Grapefruit juice, sweetened, 250 mL	0	0		485	✓
Grapefruit juice, unsweetened, 250 mL	0	0		315	✓
Grapefruit, 1/2 medium, 125g	1.0	0		140	✓
Grapefruit, canned in juice, 1/2 cup	1.0	0		150	✓
Grapefruit, canned in light syrup, 1/2 cup	1.0	0		320	✓
Grapes, black, 100g	1.0	0		265	✓✓

Food	Fibre g	Fat g	Fat Rating	Energy kJ	Carb Rating
Grapes, black, muscatel, 100g	1.0	0		330	✓✓
Grapes, green, Cornichon, 100g	1.0	0		235	✓✓
Grapes, green, sultana, 100g	1.0	0		255	✓✓
Grapes, Waltham Cross, 100g	1.0	0		255	✓✓
Grapeseed oil, 1 tbsp	0	20.0	✓✓	740	
Gravy powder, 1 tbsp, 10g	0	0		110	×
Gravy, 1/4 cup	0	5.5	××	330	×
Greek salad, average serve	2.0	25.0	✓	1080	
Greek-style yoghurt, ½ cup	0	12.0	×	750	✓
Green pawpaw, 100g	1.5	0		115	✓
Green tomato relish, 1 tbsp	0.5	0		115	
Griddle cakes (made with corn), each, 85g	1.0	6.5	×	660	✓
Griddle cakes (made with flour) each 50g	1.0	8.0	×	570	✓
Grilled cheese on toast, 1 slice, white bread	1.0	11.0	××	820	✓
Grilled cheese on toast, 1 slice, wholemeal bread	2.0	11.0	××	800	✓
Grouse, roast, weighed with bone, 125g	0	5.5	✓	600	
Guacamole, 1 tbsp	1.0	9.0	✓	360	
Guacamole, home-made, 1/4 cup	2.5	28.0	✓	1120	
Guava, 1 medium, 95g	5.0	0.5		95	✓
Guava, canned in syrup, 100g	3.2	0		260	✓
Guava, cherry-type, 10, 60g	4.0	0		70	✓
Gulab jamen, average serve,	0.5	9.0	××	675	×
Haggis, boiled, 100g	n/a	21.5	××	1290	
Halva, sesame 5 cm piece, 50g	0.5	6.0	✓✓	475	
Ham & chicken luncheon sausage, 50g	1.0	9.0	×	480	
Ham and cheese roissant,	2.0	24.5	××	1600	×
Ham steak, 1, grilled, 120g	0	9.5	×	815	
Ham, canned, leg, 50g	0	4.0	×	290	
Ham, canned, shoulder, 50g	0	3.0	×	250	
Ham, fat reduced, 97% fat free, 50g	0	1.5	×	195	

Food	Fibre g	Fat g	Fat Rating	Energy kJ	Carb Rating
Ham, leg, 50g	0	3.5	×	260	
Ham, light leg, 50g	0	2.0	×	225	
Ham, light, 90% fat-free, 50g	0	4.0	×	295	
Hamburger, Big Mac, 1	5.0	25.0	×	2010	✓
Hamburger, bun, 1, 60g	2.5	3.0	×	675	✓
Hamburger, Cheeseburger, 1	2.5	12.0	×	1190	✓
Hamburger, Junior burger, 1	2.5	8.5	×	1000	✓
Hamburger, mince, raw, 100g	0	16.0	×	925	
Hamburger, patties, home-made, 1 patty	0.5	24.0	×	1540	
Hamburger, plain, 1	3.0	18.0	×	1640	✓
Hamburger, with bacon, 1	3.0	25.0	×	2000	✓
Hamburger, with cheese, 1	3.5	26.5	×	2160	✓
Hamburger, with egg, 1	3.5	26.0	×	2170	✓
Hard sauce, 2 tbsp	0	10.0	××	960	××
Hare, casserole, average serve	0	11.5	✓	1170	
Hare, roast, average serve	0	6.0	✓	600	
Haricot beans, cooked, 1 cup, 180g	16.0	1.5	✓	680	✓✓
Haricot beans, dried, 100g	18.5	2.0	✓	1050	✓✓
Harissa, 1 tsp	0	0.5		35	
Hash browns, commercial, average serve	1.5	7.5	×	515	✓
Hash browns, home-made, 1/2 cup, 80g	1.0	11.0	×	700	✓
Hazelnut oil, 1 tbsp	0	20.0	✓✓	740	
Hazelnut torte, 1/10 of cake	2.5	31.0	××	1690	××
Hazelnuts, 50g	5.0	30.5	✓✓	1305	
Heart, lamb, 100g cooked	0	8.0	×	770	
Heart, ox, 100g cooked	0	2.5	×	625	
Heart, veal, 100g cooked	0	6.0	×	760	
Herb bread, 2 slices	2.0	32.0	××	1760	✓
Herbs, dried, mixed, 1 tbsp, 7g	0.5	0		80	
Hermesetas, granulated, ½ cup	0	0		200	
Herring, 100g can, drained, 70g	0	14.0	✓✓	610	

Food	Fibre g	Fat g	Fat Rating	Energy kJ	Carb Rating
Herrings in tomato sauce, canned, 100g	0	10.5	✓✓	735	
Hi-Fruit, frozen soft serve, 1 cone	0	0		275	×
Hokkien noodles, fresh, 100g	1.0	2.0	✓	675	✓
Hollandaise sauce, 2 tbsp	1.5	25.0	××	950	
Honey smacks, 1 cup, 40g	0.5	2.0		645	××
Honey, 1 tbsp, 25g	0	0		330	××
Honeycomb, 30g piece	0	1.5	×	360	××
Honeydew melon, 1 cup, 160g	1.5	0		210	✓
Honeydew melon, average-sized wedge, 250g	2.5	0		330	✓
Horse meat, roasted, 100g	0	6.0	×	730	
Horseradish, raw, 1 teaspoon	0.5	0		15	
Hot cakes, butter and syrup, 1 serve	2.5	10.5	××	1910	××
Hot chocolate with milk and cream, 240 mL	0	25.0	××	1500	×
Hot chocolate, made with milk, 240 mL	0	11.0	×	925	×
Hot chocolate, take-away machine, 1	0	2.0	×	400	×
Hot cross bun, 1 regular, 90g	4.5	4.0	×	1050	✓
Hot cross bun, 1 small, 45g	2.0	2.0	×	530	✓
Hot cross bun, home-made, 1	4.5	4.0	×	1280	✓
Hot dog, average	3.0	18.0	××	1445	✓
Hot fudge sundae, fast food chain, 1	0	10.5	××	1320	××
Hoummus, ¼ cup	3.5	9.5	✓✓	585	✓✓
Hoummus, lite, ¼ cup	2.0	4.5	✓✓	330	✓✓
Hoummus, supermarket brand, ¼ cup	5.5	10.0	✓✓	560	✓✓
Hungarian goulash, average serve	2.5	20.0	×	1840	
Hungry Jack Apple pie	n/a	13.0	××	1005	××
Hungry Jack Aussie Burger	n/a	32.0	×	2745	✓
Hungry Jack Bacon double cheeseburger deluxe	n/a	47.5	×	2970	✓
Hungry Jack Cheeseburger	n/a	19.5	×	1615	✓
Hungry Jack Chicken nuggets, 7 pieces	n/a	29.5	××	1725	×
Hungry Jack Cone	n/a	5.0	××	530	×
Hungry Jack Double cheeseburger	n/a	39.5	×	2715	✓

Food	Fibre g	Fat g	Fat Rating	Energy kJ	Carb Rating
Hungry Jack French fries, large, 159g	n/a	25.0	××	1975	✓
Hungry Jack French fries, regular, 114g	n/a	18.0	××	1415	✓
Hungry Jack Grilled chicken burger, 179g	n/a	27.5	×	2035	✓
Hungry Jack Ocean Catch fish sandwich	n/a	16.0	×	1640	✓
Hungry Jack Onion rings, large	n/a	19.0	××	1740	
Hungry Jack Shakes, average	0	8.0	×	1225	✓
Hungry Jack Sundaes	n/a	7.5	××	985	××
Hungry Jack Whopper Junior burger	n/a	27.5	×	1915	✓
Hungry Jack Whopper Sandwich	n/a	38.5	×	2755	✓
Hungry Jack Whopper with bacon	n/a	42.0	×	2940	✓
Hungry Jack Whopper with cheese	n/a	42.0	×	2940	✓
Hungry Jack Whopper with egg,	n/a	40.0	×	2880	✓
Hungry Jack Whopper with the lot	n/a	47.0	×	3250	✓
Ice block, frosty d-lite, 1, 100 mL	0	0.5		385	××
Ice block, frosty fruits, tropical, 1, 75mL	0	0		325	××
Ice block, Icy pole, 1, average all flavours, 75mL	0	0		200	××
Ice block, paddle pop, 1	0	3.5	×	525	××
Ice block, water, average, 1	0	0		360	××
Ice cream cone only, 5g	0	0		80	×
Ice cream cone, 2 small scoops regular, 55g	0	6.0	×	420	×
Ice cream cone, 2 small scoops rich, 110g	0	18.0	×	1115	×
Ice cream cup, 50g	0	5.0	×	390	×
Ice cream soda, 300 mL	0	2.0	×	685	××
Ice cream sugar cone, only	0	0.5		190	×
Ice cream, 3 small scoops in sugar cone	0	27.0	×	1575	×
Ice cream, Barney banana on stick, 1, 78mL	0	2.0	×	335	××
Ice cream, Billabong on stick, 1, 78mL	0	2.0	×	340	××
Ice cream, Blue Ribbon Light, 100g	0	6.0	×	755	×
Ice cream, Blue Ribbon Lite Choc, 100 mL (27g)	0	2.0	×	350	×
Ice cream, Bulla Lite Chocolate, 100 mL	0	1.0	×	270	×

Food	Fibre g	Fat g	Fat Rating	Energy kJ	Carb Rating
Ice cream, Bulla Lite Vanilla, 100 mL	0	0.5		245	×
Ice cream, butterscotch, average serve, 100 mL, 50g	0	5.5	×	465	×
Ice cream, caramel, average serve, 100 mL, 50g	0	5.5	×	410	×
Ice cream, chocolate coated heart, 1, 67g	0	14.5	××	855	×
Ice cream, chocolate coated, 1, 70g	0	15.0	××	920	×
Ice cream, chocolate, average serve, 100 mL, 50g	0	5.5	×	420	×
Ice cream, chocollo, 160g	0	0.5		705	×
Ice cream, choc-wedge, choc malt, 1, 68g	0	16.0	××	765	×
Ice cream, choc-wedge, vanilla, 1, 68g	0	17.0	××	755	×
Ice cream, Cornetto, 1, 70g	0	12.0	××	775	×
Ice cream, Dairy Bell Lite, 100 mL	0	2.0	×	235	×
Ice cream, Dairy Bell reduced fat, 100 mL	0	2.5	×	270	×
Ice cream, deep-fried, average serve	2	35.0	××	2500	××
Ice cream, Drumstick, average, 1, 75g	0	16.5	××	900	××
Ice cream, Fruit de Light on stick, 1, 78mL	0	0.5		220	××
Ice cream, Gaytime, 1, 67g	0	12.0	××	755	××
Ice cream, Gelati Italia, chocolate, 100g serve	0	7.0	×	700	×
Ice cream, Gelati Italia, hazelnut, 100g serve	0	6.5	×	805	×
Ice cream, Gelati Italia, lemon sorbet, 100g serve	0	1.5	×	480	×
Ice cream, Gelati Italia, mango, 100g serve	0	1.5	×	485	×
Ice cream, Heart,1, 77g	0	20.5	××	935	××
Ice cream, Neapolitan, average serve, 100 mL, 50g	0	5.5	×	415	×
Ice cream, Norco, Light Slice, 1, 45g	0	1.0	×	250	×
Ice cream, Norco, Prestige, Light, Peach, 100 mL	0	1.0	×	260	×
Ice cream, Norco, Prestige, Light, Toffee, 100 mL	0	1.5	×	315	×
Ice cream, Norco, Slice, 1, 45g	0	1.5	×	735	×

Food	Fibre g	Fat g	Fat Rating	Energy kJ	Carb Rating
Ice cream, one-whip, home-made, 2 scoops	0	5.0	×	405	×
Ice cream, Peters Light & Creamy slices, 1, 51g	0	1.5	×	305	×
Ice cream, Peters Light & Creamy slices, choc, 1, 73g	0	2.0	×	515	×
Ice cream, Peters Light & Creamy, chocolate swirl, 100g	0	3.0	×	660	×
Ice cream, Peters Light & Creamy, chocolate, 100g	0	3.0	×	620	×
Ice cream, Peters Light & Creamy, passionfruit, 100g	0	3.0	×	685	×
Ice cream, Peters Light & Creamy, vanilla, 100g	0	3.0	×	615	×
Ice cream, Peters Light & Creamy, vanilla, 100g	0	3.0	×	615	×
Ice cream, Peters, Royal chocolate, 100g	0	12.0	××	875	×
Ice cream, polyunsaturated, average serve, 50g	0	5.0	✓	390	×
Ice cream, rich home-made, 2 scoops	0	34.0	××	1500	×
Ice cream, Sara Lee, Butterscothc, 70g (100mL)	0	11.0	×	845	×
Ice cream, Sara Lee, Classic Lite, 60g (100 mL)	0	4.5	×	540	×
Ice cream, So Good mango, 100g	0	2.0	✓	460	×
Ice cream, soft serve, frozen, Gise, 100mL	0	0		125	×
Ice cream, soft serve, frozen, Just 10, 100mL	0	0		125	
Ice cream, soft serve, frozen, Just Trim, 100mL	0	3.0	×	330	×
Ice cream, soft serve, small cone	0	2.5	×	470	×
Ice cream, split, pine-lime, on stick, 1, 63g	0	4.0	×	340	××
Ice cream, split, raspberry, on stick, 1, 62g	0	2.5	×	265	××
Ice cream, strawberry vanilla yoghurt, 1, 78g	0	0		280	×
Ice cream, Streets light vanilla, 2 small scoops, 65g	0	4.0	×	490	×
Ice cream, sundae, hot fudge, cream & nuts, 1	1.0	59.0	××	3000	××
Ice cream, vanilla light slice, 1, 100 mL	0	1.5	×	305	×
Ice cream, vanilla, average serve, 100 mL, 50g	0	5.0	×	415	×
Ice cream, Vitari, 100 mL	0	0		235	×
Ice cream, Weight Watchers, chocolate, 145 mL	0	0.5		420	×

Food	Fibre g	Fat g	Fat Rating	Energy kJ	Carb Rating
Ice cream, Weight Watchers, mango, 145 mL	0	0.5		540	✗
Ice cream, Weight Watchers, vanilla, 145 mL	0	0.5		410	✗
Ice cream, with fruit & nuts, 70g	0	6.0	✗	500	✗
Ice cream, with yoghurt, Alfresko, 1, 180 mL	0	4.0	✗	595	✗
Ice cream, wrapped cone, 70g	0	11.0	✗✗	810	✗
Ice dessert, tofu, low fat, 100g	0	4.0	✗	515	✗
Ice dessert, tofu, soft serve, average, 110g	0	8.0	✗	660	✗
Iced chocolate, 250 mL	0	25.0	✗	1680	✗
Iced coffee, café, average serve	0	23.0	✗	1255	✗
Iced coffee, carton, 300 mL	0	10.0	✗	955	✗
Icy Pole, 1, 75mL	0	0		190	✗✗
Indian fresh cheese, 50g	0	11.0	✗	780	
Indian seasoning, Cuisine Essentials, 1 tbsp	0	0		80	
Instant porridge, 1 sachet	2.5	2.0	✓✓	470	✓✓
Irish coffee, 200 mL	0	11.0	✗✗	855	
Irish moss, (seaweed), raw, 2 tbsp, 10g	0	0		20	
Irish potato cakes, 1, 50g	1.0	8.0	✗✗	500	✓
Irish soda bread, 1/10 25cm loaf	4.5	7.0	✗✗	1275	✓
Irish stew, average serve, 350g	3.5	22.0	✗	1560	✓
Italian dressing, 1 tbsp	0	6.5	✓	260	
Italian dressing, reduced fat, 1 tbsp	0	0		25	
Jackfruit, flesh only, 100g	3.0	0		325	✓
Jam sponge roll, 1 slice, 50g	0.5	1.0	✗	605	✗✗
Jam tart, 1 small, 50g	0.5	7.5	✗✗	745	✗✗
Jam, any type, 1 tbsp, 20g	0	0		210	✗
Jam, fruit spread, no added sugar, 1 tbsp, 20g	0.5	0		140	✗
Jambalaya, average serve	4.0	26.0	✗	2690	✓
Jarlsberg, see cheese					
Jatz crackers, 6, 25g	0.5	5.0	✗✗	460	✗
Jelly beans, 30g	0	0		420	✗✗
Jelly snakes, 30g	0	0		420	✗✗

Food	Fibre g	Fat g	Fat Rating	Energy kJ	Carb Rating
Jelly, average serve, (1/4 packet),125g	0	0		355	××
Jerusalem artichoke, 100g	3.0	0		100	✓✓
Jewfish, grilled, 150g	0	1.0	✓✓	540	
Jicama (vegetable), 1 cup, 120g	6.0	0		190	✓
John dory fish, grilled, 150g	0	1.0	✓✓	570	
Juice drink, apple, 35% juice, 250 mL	0	0		425	×
Juice drink, apricot, 250 mL	0	0		570	×
Juice drink, orange & mango, 250 mL	0	0		565	×
Juice drink, orange, 250 mL	0	0		515	×
Juice fruit drink, apple, 250 mL	0	0		425	✓
Juice fruit drink, orange & mango, 250 mL	0	0		405	✓
Juice fruit drink, orange, 250 mL	0	0		405	✓
Juice fruit drink, tropical, 250 mL	0	0		390	✓
Juice, apple, carbonated, 250 mL	0	0		435	××
Juice, apple, no sugar, 250 mL	0	0		440	✓
Juice, grape, dark, 250 mL	0	0		590	✓
Juice, grape, unsweetened, 250 mL	0	0		490	✓
Juice, grapefruit, unsweetened, 250 mL	0	0		315	✓
Juice, lemon, 1 tbsp	0	0		5	
Juice, lime, 1 tbsp	0	0		5	
Juice, orange & mango, 250 mL	0	0		565	✓
Juice, orange, 250 mL	0	0		380	✓
Juice, orange, no sugar, 250 mL	0	0		355	✓
Juice, pineapple, unsweetened, 250 mL	0	0		490	✓
Juice, tomato, canned, 250 mL	2.0	0		200	✓
Juice, vegetable, canned, 250 mL	2.0	0		150	
Junior burger, 1	3.0	8.0	×	1020	✓
Junket, average serve	0	5.0	×	380	✓
Just Right, 1 cup, 60g	5.5	1.5	✓	890	✓
Kabana sausage, 50g	0	12.5	×	585	
Kalamata olives, marinated, 20g	1.0	5.5g	✓	225	

Food	Fibre g	Fat g	Fat Rating	Energy kJ	Carb Rating
Kalamata olives, mixed, brine, 20g	1.0	0.5g	✓	90	
Kalamata olives, plain, in oil, 20g	1.0	6.5g	✓	315	
Kale, cooked, 1/2 cup, 65g	1.5	0.5		65	
Kale, raw, 1/2 cup shredded, 35g	1.0	0.5		50	
Kangaroo mettwurst, 50g	0	2.0	✓	315	
Kangaroo, rump, 125g	0	2.5	✓	620	
Kantong noodles, 99% fat free, 200g	4.5	1.0	×	1010	✓
Kataifi, Greek pastry, 1, 125g	1.0	12.0	××	1560	××
Kebab, doner, 1	8.0	24.0	×	2500	✓
Kecap manis, 1 tbsp	0	0		365	×
Kedgeree, average serve, 200g	0.5	16.0	✓	1400	✓
Kelp (seaweed), raw, 10g	0	0		20	
KFC bacon & cheese chicken fillet burger, 1, 193g	1.0	26.0	×	2065	✓
KFC bean salad, 100g	3.5	5.0	✓	565	✓✓
KFC Chips, large	9.0	34.0	××	2500	✓
KFC Chips, regular	4.5	17.5	××	1185	✓
KFC Coleslaw, 100g	3.5	4.0	✓	400	
KFC Colonel burger, 1, 114g	0.5	14.5	×	1195	✓
KFC fried chicken, average piece	0	15.0	×	900	✓
KFC Mashed potato & gravy, 100g	0.5	2.0	×	280	✓
KFC Nuggets, 6, 108g	0.5	17.5	××	995	×
KFC Potato salad, 100g	1.0	6.5	×	560	✓
KFC Works burger, 1, 233g	1.5	26.0	×	2180	✓
KFC, bacon & cheese chicken fillet burger, 1	n/a	22.5	×	1930	✓
KFC, bacon & cheese zinger burger, 1	n/a	18.5	×	2045	✓
KFC, cheesecake, 1	n/a	7.0	××	735	××
KFC, chicken fillet burger, 1, 170g	1.0	22.5	×	1785	✓
KFC, fried chicken, breast, 1 piece	0	14.5	×	1020	
KFC, fried chicken, drumstick, 1 piece	0	4.0	×	560	
KFC, fried chicken, rib, 1 piece	0	15.5	×	955	

Food	Fibre g	Fat g	Fat Rating	Energy kJ	Carb Rating
KFC, fried chicken, thigh, 1 piece	0	22.5	×	1200	
KFC, fried chicken, wing, 1 piece	0	10.5	×	570	
KFC, gravy, ¼ cup	0	5.5	××	265	
KFC, Stuffing, 2 tbsps	0.5	2.0	××	200	×
Kibbeh, vegetarian, 4 small	9.5	16.0	✓✓	1270	✓✓
Kibbeh, with lamb, average serve, 4 small	9.5	17.0	✓	1590	✓✓
Kidney beans, canned, ½ cup, 95g	6.0	0.5		340	✓✓
Kidney beans, canned, drained, ½ cup, 100g	6.5	0.5		360	✓✓
Kidney beans, cooked, 1 cup, 185g	20.0	0.5		890	✓✓
Kidney beans, dried, ½ cup, 95g	10.5	0.5		455	✓✓
Kidney, lamb, 2 cooked, 80g	0	3.5	×	490	
Kidney, ox, cooked, 100g	0	2.5	×	565	
Kidney, veal, cooked, 100g	0	6.5	×	700	
Kidneys in mustard cream sauce, average serve	0	35.0	×	1890	
Kingfish, grilled, 150g	0	1.0	✓✓	585	
Kipper, baked, 100g	0	6.0	✓✓	465	
Kit Kat bar, 1 45g	0	11.0	××	940	××
Kit Kat chunky bar, 1 60g	0	18.0	××	1330	××
Kiwi fruit, 1 average, 90g	3.0	0		185	✓
Koftas, average serve, 175g	1.5	48.0	××	2570	✓
Kohl rabi, (cabbage turnip), cooked, 75g	3.0	0		115	✓
Kombu, (seaweed), dried, raw, 10g	6.0	0		20	
Komplete muesli, 1/2 cup, 60g	4.5	5.5	×	975	✓✓
Korma curry sauce, packet, made up, ½ cup	1.0	18.0	✓	920	×
Korma spices, Charmaine Solomon, 25g	1.0	5.0	✓	255	
Kulfi (Indian ice cream), average serve	3.0	29.0	×	2500	✓
Kumara, 100g baked	3.0	0		420	✓
Kurrajong pod, 100g	n/a	0		1290	✓
Lady's fingers (filo, meat, onion, pine nuts), 1, 40g	0.5	7.0	✓	475	×
Laksa curry paste, 1 tbsp	0.5	0.5		80	

Food	Fibre g	Fat g	Fat Rating	Energy kJ	Carb Rating
Laksa, average bowl	3.5	22.0	××	1600	✓
Lamb butterfly steak, raw, 100g	0	4.5	×	525	
Lamb rissoles, cheese & honey, 2, 150g	0	23.0	×	1390	
Lamb strips, raw, 100g	0	6.0	×	565	
Lamb, boneless, lean cuts, 150g	0	5.5	×	760	
Lamb, breast, rolled, stuffed, baked, 2 slices, 100g	0	21.5	×	1210	
Lamb, chump chop, grilled, lean & fat, 2	0	24.0	×	1540	
Lamb, chump chop, grilled, lean only, 2	0	9.0	×	945	
Lamb, cutlet, crumbed, 2	0.5	17.5	×	980	
Lamb, cutlet, grilled or baked, lean & fat, 2	0	21.5	×	1110	
Lamb, cutlet, grilled or baked, lean only, 2	0	5.0	×	470	
Lamb, Easy carve leg, cooked, 100g	0	7.5	×	760	
Lamb, French rack or cutlets, baked, lean, 3	0	9.0	×	690	
Lamb, kebabs, satay sauce, 2 sticks	0	30.0	×	1880	
Lamb, Korma, average serve, 200g	2.0	18.0	×	1490	
Lamb, leg, baked, lean & fat, 2 slices, 90g	0	10.5	×	845	
Lamb, leg, baked, lean only, 2 slices, 80g	0	4.5	×	600	
Lamb, loin chop, grilled, lean & fat, 2	0	30.0	×	1470	
Lamb, loin chop, grilled, lean only, 2	0	5.0	×	500	
Lamb, neck chop, stewed, lean & fat, 1	0	14.0	×	740	
Lamb, neck chop, stewed, lean only, 1	0	5.5	×	425	
Lamb, shank, cooked, lean & fat, 1	0	8.5	×	875	
Lamb, shank, cooked, lean only, 1	0	4.0	×	655	
Lamb, shoulder, baked, lean & fat, 2 slices, 80g	0	12.0	×	825	
Lamb, shoulder, baked, lean only, 2 slices, 80g	0	5.5	×	625	
Lamb, tandoori, 200g	0.5	38.0	×	2210	✓
Lamb, tongue, canned, 100g	0	14.0	×	810	
Lamb, topside roast, lean, baked, 100g	0	5.5	×	745	
Lamb, topside, raw, 100g	0	4.5	×	530	
Lamb, Trim, boneless loin, roast, 100g	0	8.5	×	810	

Food	Fibre g	Fat g	Fat Rating	Energy kJ	Carb Rating
Lamb, Trim, butterfly steak, raw, 100g	0	4.5	×	525	
Lamb, Trim, fillet, raw, 100g	0	4.0	×	485	
Lamb, Trim, schnitzel steak, cooked, 120g	0	5.5	×	775	
Lamb, Trim, strips, raw, 100g	0	3.5	×	480	
Lambs lettuce, raw, 1/2 cup	1.0	0		70	
Lamington, average cake-shop, 1, 75g	1.5	9.0	××	980	××
Lamington, home-made, 1, 60g	1.0	6.0	××	815	××
Lamington, packet, 1, 50g	1.0	6.0	××	655	××
Lard, 100g	0	100.0	××	7400	
Lasagne sheets, dry, 3 sheets, 50g	1.5	0.5		770	✓✓
Lasagne sheets, fresh, 1 large sheet, 150g	3.0	1.5	✓	1160	✓✓
Lasagne, frozen, 300g	9.0	17.0	×	1630	✓✓
Lasagne, frozen, lite, chicken & vegetable, 300g	n/a	9.0	×	1260	✓✓
Lasagne, frozen, lite, ricotta & spinach, 300g	n/a	14.5	×	1260	✓✓
Lasagne, home-made with ricotta, average serve	3.0	30.0	×	2330	✓✓
Lasagne, home-made, average serve	5.5	23.0	×	2630	✓✓
Lasagne, restaurant, average serve	6.0	48.0	×	3880	✓
Lasagne, take-away, entree, 210g	3.0	8.0	×	925	✓
Lasagne, take-away, main course, 350g	5.0	13.5	×	1545	✓
Lasagne, vegetarian, restaurant, average serve	11.0	29.0	×	2600	✓✓
Lavash bread, 1 slice, 56g	2.0	1.5	✓	690	✓
Laver (seaweed), canned, 100g	34.0	0		115	
Laver (seaweed), raw, 10 sheets	0.5	0		40	
Le Snak (biscuits & cheese spread),1, 25g	0.5	6.5	××	400	×
Leather jacket, steamed, 150g	0	0.5	✓	525	
Lebanese cucumber, 1 average, 130g	1.5	0		65	
Leben, (yoghurt) 200g	0	6.5	×	660	✓
Lecithin, soy, 1 tbsp, 10g	1.5	6.0	✓	250	
Leek and potato soup, 1 cup, 250g	1.5	6.0	×	450	✓
Leek, 1 whole, 125g	3.5	0.5		125	
Leek, sliced, 1/2 cup raw, 45g	1.5	0		50	

Food	Fibre g	Fat g	Fat Rating	Energy kJ	Carb Rating
Leek, sliced, cooked in oil, 1/2 cup, 80g	2.5	10.5	✓	80	
Lemon butter, home-made, 1 tbsp	0	4.0	×	300	××
Lemon crush, frozen, 100 mL	0	0		105	××
Lemon curd, commercial, 1 tbsp	0	1.0	×	240	××
Lemon delicious pudding, average serve	0.5	11.0	××	995	××
Lemon flavour soft drink, 1 can, 370 mL	0	0		735	××
Lemon juice, 1 tbsp	0	0		5	
Lemon meringue pie, 1/6 23 cm pie	0.5	18.0	××	1850	××
Lemon meringue pie. Home-made, 1/8 23 cm pie	1.0	12.0	××	1300	××
Lemon sole, grilled, 150g	0	2.0	✓✓	515	
Lemon sorbet, 100g	0	1.5	×	485	××
Lemon tart, average serve	1.5	22.0	××	1900	××
Lemon, fresh, 1 medium, including skin 100g	4.5	0		80	
Lemon, fresh, 1 medium, without skin, 65g	1.5	0		55	
Lemonade, 1 glass, 250 mL	0	0		440	××
Lemongrass, 1 stalk, crushed	1.5	0		40	
Lentil burger patty, 1 average	7.0	3.0	✓	1100	✓✓
Lentil sprouts, 1/2 cup, 30g	0.5	0		130	
Lentils, brown or green, 1/2 cup dry, 95g	8.5	2.0	✓✓	1200	✓✓
Lentils, brown or green, cooked, 1 cup, 190g	7.0	1.5	✓✓	845	✓✓
Lentils, red, cooked, 1 cup, 190g	6.5	1.0	✓✓	805	✓✓
Lentils, red, dry, 1/2 cup, 100g	10.5	1.5	✓✓	1355	✓✓
Lettuce, cos, 2 leaves	0.5	0		15	
Lettuce, iceberg, 2 leaves	0.5	0		10	
Lettuce, mignonette, 2 leaves	0.5	0		10	
Lettuce, radicchio, 2 leaves	0.5	0		15	
Lilli-pilli, 10 average	2.0	0		95	
Lima beans cooked, 1 cup, 180g	8.5	1.0	✓✓	785	✓✓
Lima beans, canned, drained, 1 cup, 220g	10.0	1.0	✓✓	720	✓✓
Lima beans, dried, uncooked, 1/2 cup, 90g	18.0	1.5	✓✓	1110	✓✓

Food	Fibre g	Fat g	Fat Rating	Energy kJ	Carb Rating
Lime juice, 1 tbsp	0	0		5	
Lime, 1/4 lime	0.5	0		20	
Ling fish, grilled, 150g	0	0.5	✓✓	590	
Linseeds, 1 tbsp, 10g	3.0	2.5	✓✓	190	
Liqueur, advocaat, 1 glass, 40 mL	0	0		455	×
Liqueur, coffee, 1 glass, 40 mL	0	0		660	×
Liqueur, cointreau, 1 glass, 40 mL	0	0		525	×
Liqueur, curacao, 1 glass, 40 mL	0	0		520	×
Liquorice allsorts, 3, 24g	0	0.5		170	××
Liquorice, 50g	1.5	0.5		480	××
Liquorice, raspberry, 50g	1.0	0.5		660	××
Lite Bix, 2 biscuits, 30g	3.5	1.0	✓	400	✓
Lite 'n' tasty, 1 cup, 45g	1.0	0		670	✓
Lite Start Plus, 1 cup, 45g	2.0	0		720	✓
Liver, calves, raw, 100g	0	5.5	×	580	
Liver, lamb, raw, 100g	0	7.5	×	680	
Liver, lamb's fry with bacon, 150g	0	21.5	×	1850	
Liver, ox, raw, 100g	0	8.5	×	655	
Liverwurst, 50g	0.5	14.0	×	690	
Lobster, 100g	0	1.0	✓✓	360	
Lobster, Asian style, 150g	0.5	10.0	✓✓	840	
Loganberries, 100g	6.5	0		110	✓✓
Lollies, boiled, 4, 15g	0	0		195	××
Longans, fresh, 10, 30g	0.5	0		75	✓
Loquats, 6 medium, 60g	1.0	0		65	✓
Lotus root, canned, 10 slices, 85g	0.5	0		50	
Lotus root, raw, 1/2 root, 60g	1.0	0		110	✓
Lotus seeds, dried, 1/2 cup, 16g	n/a	0.5		225	✓
LSA mix, 2 tbsp	4.5	8.5	✓✓	450	
Lucozade drink, 250 mL	0	0		720	××
Luffa, angled (long okra), 75g	1.0	0		40	

Food	Fibre g	Fat g	Fat Rating	Energy kJ	Carb Rating
Lychees, canned, 1 cup	1.5	0		710	✓
Lychees, fresh, 6 average, 60g	1.0	0		170	✓
M&Ms peanut, 55g	2.5	13.5	××	1145	××
M&Ms, 55g	1.5	10.5	××	1080	××
Macadamia nut oil, 1 tbsp	0	20.0	✓✓	740	
Macadamia nuts, 50g	3.0	38.0	✓✓	1510	
Macaroni cheese, home-made, 230g	2.0	34.0	×	2540	✓
Macaroni cheese, Snack stop, 1 serve	n/a	8.0	×	1430	✓
Macaroni, cooked, 1 cup	2.0	1.0	✓	550	✓✓
Macaroni, dry, 1 cup	4.5	1.5	✓	1335	✓✓
Macaroons, almond, home-made, 1	1.0	6.0	×	540	×
Mackerel, smoked, 75g	0	23.0	✓✓	1100	
Madeira cake, small slice, 60g	0.5	9.0	××	930	××
Maitre d'hotel butter, 15g	0	2.0	××	175	
Maize oil, 1 tbsp	0	20.0	✓✓	740	
Malted milk powder, 1 tbsp, 10g	0	0.5		160	✓
Maltesers, 45g	1.0	9.5	××	890	××
Mandarin oranges, canned, 100g	0.5	0		225	✓
Mandarin, 1 large	2.5	0		175	✓
Mandarins, Clementines, each	1.5	0		120	✓
Mange-tout peas, 50g	2.0	0		80	✓
Mango chutney, oily, 1 tbsp	0.5	2.0	✓	240	×
Mango chutney, sweet, 1 tbsp	0.5	0		160	×
Mango, 1 large, 430g	8.5	0.5		715	✓
Mango, 1 medium, 250g	5.0	0		415	✓
Mango, green, 1/2 medium, 125g	3.0	0		245	✓
Maple syrup, 1 tbsp	0	0		220	××
Margarine, canola, 1 tbsp	0	14.0	✓✓	520	
Margarine, cooking, 1 tbsp	0	16.0	××	600	
Margarine, fat-reduced Becel Diet, 1 tbsp	0	8.0	✓	305	
Margarine, fat-reduced Flora light, 1 tbsp	0	10.0	✓	370	

Food	Fibre g	Fat g	Fat Rating	Energy kJ	Carb Rating
Margarine, Flora canola, 1 tbsp	0	16.0	✓	600	
Margarine, Gold 'n Canola lite, 1 tbsp	0	12.0	✓✓	440	
Margarine, Gold 'n Canola, 1 tbsp	0	14.0	✓✓	520	
Margarine, I Can't Believe It's Not Butter, 1 tbsp	0	16.0	✓	590	
Margarine, Logicol, 1 tbsp	0	13.5	✓✓	495	
Margarine, Meadowlea Lite, 1 tbsp	0	12.0	✓✓	430	
Margarine, Meadowlea Milk free, 1 tbsp	0	15.0	✓✓	555	
Margarine, Meadowlea Original, 1 tbsp	0	15.0	✓	555	
Margarine, Miracle canola, 1 tbsp	0	13.0	✓✓	475	
Margarine, monounsaturated, 1 tbsp	0	16.0	✓	590	
Margarine, Nuttelex, 1 tbsp	0	16.5	✓	615	
Margarine, Olive Grove Classic/Extra virgin, 1 tbsp	0	15.0	✓✓	555	
Margarine, Olive Grove Lite, 1 tbsp	0	12.0	✓	440	
Margarine, Olivio, 1 tbsp	0	15.0	✓✓	555	
Margarine, Olivio, Light, 1 tbsp	0	12.0	✓	435	
Margarine, polyunsaturated, 1 tbsp	0	16.0	✓	590	
Margarine, ProActiv, 1 tbsp	0	13.0	✓	480	
Margarine, table, 1 tbsp	0	16.0	××	600	
Marinara sauce (for pasta), no cream, average serve	1.0	3.0	✓	645	
Marmalade, 1 tbsp	0	0		210	××
Marmalade, home-made, 1 tbsp	0.5	0		130	×
Marmite, 1 tsp	0	0		25	
Marrow, 100g	1.0	0		40	
Mars almond bar, 1, 50g	1.5	12.5	××	1150	××
Mars bar, 63g	1.0	11.0	××	1090	××
Mars bar, Lite, 1, 45g	0.5	5.5	×	800	××
Marshmallows, 50g	0	0		675	××
Marshmallows, chocolate, 50g	0	5.5	×	850	××
Marshmallows, coconut, 1	0.5	0.5		225	××
Marshmallows, home-made, each	0	0		260	××

Food	Fibre g	Fat g	Fat Rating	Energy kJ	Carb Rating
Martini	0	0		505	
Marzipan, home-made, 30g	1.5	7.5	✓	580	××
Marzipan, purchased, 30g	1.0	4.5	✓	510	××
Mascarpone, 30g	0	14.0	××	555	
Mayonnaise, 90% fat-free, 1 tbsp	0	2.0	✓	140	
Mayonnaise, 97% fat-free, 1 tbsp	0	0.5		110	
Mayonnaise, commercial, 1 tbsp	0	6.5	✓	310	
Mayonnaise, Heinz traditional, 1 tbsp	0	8.5	✓	360	
Mayonnaise, Hellman's light, 1 tbsp	0	6.5	✓	280	
Mayonnaise, home-made, 1 tbsp	0	18.0	✓	665	
Mayonnaise, Praise no cholesterol, 1 tbsp, 20g	0	7.0	✓	310	
Mayonnaise, reduced fat, 1 tbsp	0	4.0	✓	240	
McDonald's, Apple pie, 1	1.5	18.5	××	1250	××
McDonald's, Bacon & Egg McMuffin, 1	2.0	15.0	×	1300	✓
McDonald's, Barbecue sauce, 1 portion	0	0.5		180	×
McDonald's, Berry Nice Yoghurt Crunch, 1	2.5	4.5	×	960	×
McDonald's, Big breakfast	3.5	30.0	×	2200	✓
McDonald's, Big Mac, 1	5.0	25.0	×	2010	✓
McDonald's, cappuccino, large, 1	0	0		315	✓
McDonald's, cappuccino, regular, 1	0	0		245	✓
McDonald's, Cheese & tomato sandwich, 1	2.5	5.5	×	950	✓
McDonald's, Cheeseburger, 1	2.5	12.0	×	1190	✓
McDonald's, Chicken Caesar salad, 1	n/a	7.5	×	950	✓
McDonald's, Chicken foldover, 1	2.5	9.0	×	1480	✓
McDonald's, Cookies, 1	1.5	8.0	×	1170	××
McDonald's, English muffin & jam, 1	2.0	4.5	×	850	✓
McDonald's, Fillet-o-fish, 1	2.0	14.0	×	1350	×
McDonald's, French fries, large	6.0	24.5	××	2010	✓
McDonald's, French fries, medium	4.5	18.0	××	1450	✓
McDonald's, French fries, regular	3.5	13.5	××	1110	✓
McDonald's, Hash browns	1.5	7.5	×	515	✓

Food	Fibre g	Fat g	Fat Rating	Energy kJ	Carb Rating
McDonald's, Hot cakes, butter and syrup, 1 serve	2.5	10.5	××	1910	×
McDonald's, Hot cakes, no butter or syrup, 1 serve	2.5	1.0	××	810	×
McDonald's, Hot chocolate, 1	0.5	2.0	×	380	×
McDonald's, Junior burger, 1	2.5	8.5	×	1000	✓
McDonald's, McChicken, 1	4.0	22.0	×	1830	✓
McDonalds, McFlurry Crunchie, 1	0	16.0	××	1780	××
McDonald's, McFlurry M&M Mini, 1	1.0	17.5	××	1970	××
McDonald's, McFlurry Oreo cookie, 1	0.5	14.0	××	1650	××
McDonald's, McNuggets, 6 piece	0.5	20.5	××	1350	×
McDonald's, McOz, 1	4.5	30.5	×	2080	✓
McDonald's, Muffin, apple, blueberry, 1	2.5	2.5	✓	1190	×
McDonald's, Muffin, orange, poppyseed, 1	2.0	3.5	✓	1400	××
McDonald's, Quarter pounder with cheese, 1	4.5	33.5	×	2270	✓
McDonald's, Roast Chicken salad, 1	4.0	6.5	×	945	×
McDonald's, Salad, Garden, 1	2.5	4.0	✓	310	
McDonald's, Sausage McMuffin with egg, 1	2.05	17.5	×	1420	✓
McDonald's, Sausage McMuffin, 1	2.0	13.0	×	1200	✓
McDonald's, Scrambled egg McMuffin, 1	3.5	16.5	×	1405	✓
McDonald's, Shake, chocolate, large	2.0	14.0	×	2200	×
McDonald's, Shake, chocolate, medium	1.5	10.0	×	1600	×
McDonald's, Shake, strawberry, vanilla, medium	0	9.5	×	1550	×
McDonald's, Sundae cone, 1	0	4.5	×	605	×
McDonald's, Sundae, hot caramel	0	9.0	××	1430	××
McDonald's, Sundae, hot fudge, 1	1.0	12.0	××	1440	××
McDonald's, Sundae, no topping, 1	0	7.0	××	855	××
McDonald's, Sundae, strawberry, 1	0.5	7.0	××	1170	××
McDonald's, Vegeburger, 1	8.0	10.0	✓	1705	✓✓
Meat paste, 1 teaspoon	0	0.5		35	
Meat pie, 1, 175g	2.0	24.0	××	1660	×
Meat pie, home-made, average serve	1.5	36.0	×	2500	×

Food	Fibre g	Fat g	Fat Rating	Energy kJ	Carb Rating
Meat pie, lite, 175g	2.0	11.0	××	1510	×
Meat pie, party size, 50g	0.5	9.5	××	580	×
Meatballs, average serve, 230g	1.5	19.0	×	1625	
Meatloaf, 1 slice	1.0	28.0	×	2140	
Melba toast, 6 slices, 20g	0.5	0.5		325	✓
Melon, bitter (balsam pear or foo gwa), 100g	1.5	0		20	
Melon, casaba, 1 cup cubed, 160g	1.5	0		175	✓
Melon, casaba, 1 slice, 150g	1.5	0		165	✓
Melon, hairy (vegetable), 100g	1.5	0		45	
Melon, honeydew, 1 cup cubed, 160g	1.5	0		210	✓
Melon, honeydew, average-sized wedge, 250g	2.5	0		330	✓
Melon, rock, ¼ medium, 250g	2.5	0		230	✓
Melon, rock, 1 cup cubed, 160g	1.5	0		145	✓
Melon, water, 1 cup cubed, 160g	1.0	0		155	✓
Melon, water, 1 slice, 250g	1.0	0		240	✓
Meringue, commercial, each, 25g	0	0.5		385	××
Meringues, home-made, each small	0	0		115	××
Mexican spice, Cuisine Essentials, 1 tbsp	0	0		80	
Milk, Balance high calcium, 1 cup, 250 mL	0	0.5		485	✓
Milk, buffalo, 1 cup, 250 mL	0	17.0	×	1010	✓
Milk, Diploma calcium rich skim, 1 cup, 250 mL	0	0		365	✓
Milk, Diploma reduced fat light, 1 cup, 250 mL	0	0		520	✓
Milk, evaporated, canned, ½ cup, 125 mL	0	10.5	×	820	✓
Milk, evaporated, reduced-fat/canned, ½ cup, 125mL	0	2.0	×	500	✓
Milk, evaporated, skim, canned, ½ cup, 125 mL	0	0.5		395	✓
Milk, Farmers Best with omega 3, 250 mL	0	3.5	✓✓	635	✓
Milk, Farmers Best, 250 mL	0	3.5	✓	575	✓
Milk, fat-reduced UHT, 1 cup, 250 mL	0	3.0	×	520	✓
Milk, fat-reduced, protein increased, 1 cup, 250 mL	0	4.5	×	565	✓

Food	Fibre g	Fat g	Fat Rating	Energy kJ	Carb Rating
Milk, Fit 4, 1 cup, 250 mL	0	2.5	×	510	✓
Milk, flavoured reduced fat, chocolate, 300 mL	0	5.0	×	760	✓
Milk, flavoured reduced fat, strawberry, 300 mL	0	4.5	×	775	✓
Milk, flavoured, chocolate, 300 mL	0	11.0	×	995	✓
Milk, flavoured, strawberry, 300 mL	0	10.5	×	975	✓
Milk, full-cream, 1 cup, 250 mL	0	9.5	×	675	✓
Milk, full-cream, in tea or coffee, 20 mL	0	0.5		55	✓
Milk, goat's, 1 cup, 250 mL	0	8.5	×	700	✓
Milk, human, colostrum, 100g	0	2.5	✓	235	✓
Milk, human, mature, 100g	0	4.0	✓	290	✓
Milk, human, transitional, 100g	0	3.5	✓	280	✓
Milk, Lite Start, 1 cup, 250 mL	0	3.5	×	550	✓
Milk, Lite White, 1 cup, 250 mL	0	3.5	×	550	✓
Milk, powdered skim, instant, 25g	0	0		370	✓
Milk, powdered, full cream, 2 tbsp, 15g	0	4.0	×	305	✓
Milk, powdered, skim, 2 tbsp, 15g	0	0		220	✓
Milk, Pura, Edge, 1 cup, 250 mL	0	2.5	×	485	✓
Milk, Pura, Light Start, 1 cup, 250 mL	0	2.5	×	495	✓
Milk, reduced-fat, calcium enriched, 1 cup, 250 mL	0	2.5	×	485	✓
Milk, Rev, 250 mL	0	3.0	×	520	✓
Milk, shake, average, 250 mL	0	8.0	×	950	✓
Milk, Shape, 1 cup, 250 mL	0	0.5		505	✓
Milk, sheep's, 1 cup, 250 mL	0	16.5	××	1070	✓
Milk, skim, 1 cup, 250 mL	0	0		365	✓
Milk, skimmer, fat-reduced, 1 cup, 250 mL	0	4.5	×	505	✓
Milk, Smart, 1 cup, 250 mL	0	3.0	×	520	✓
Milk, soy, fortified, 1 cup, 250 mL	0	8.0	✓	650	✓
Milk, soy, fortified, flavoured, 1 cup, 250 mL	0	8.0	✓	800	✓
Milk, soy, Good Life, 1 cup, 250 mL	0	2.5	✓	450	✓
Milk, soy, lite, 1 cup, 250 mL	0	2.5	✓	460	✓

Food	Fibre g	Fat g	Fat Rating	Energy kJ	Carb Rating
Milk, soy, low fat, fortified, 1 cup, 250 mL	0	1.5	✓	450	✓
Milk, soy, So Good Fat free, 250 mL	0	0		400	✓
Milk, soy, So Good Lite, 250 mL	0	1.5	✓	450	✓
Milk, soy, So Good Smoothie, 250 mL	0	4.0	✓	750	✓
Milk, soy, So Good, 250 mL	0	8.5	✓	650	✓
Milk, soy, Soy Life, 1 cup, 250 mL	0	8.5	✓	715	✓
Milk, soy, Soy Life, low-fat, 1 cup, 250 mL	0	2.5	✓	475	✓
Milk, soy, unfortified, 1 cup, 250 mL	0	5.5	✓	410	✓
Milk, sweetened condensed, ½ cup, 150g	0	11.5	×	1715	×
Milk, sweetened condensed, 1 tbsp, 25g	0	2.0	×	345	×
Milk, sweetened condensed, skim, ½ cup, 150g	0	0.5		1415	×
Milk, sweetened condensed, skim, 1 tbsp, 25g	0	0		300	×
Milk, Take Care, low fat, 1 cup, 250 mL	0	2.5	×	485	✓
Milk, Tone, 1 cup 250 mL	0	0		490	✓
Milk, Trim, 1 cup, 250 mL	0	4.0	×	480	✓
Milk, Vaalia low-fat dairy, flavoured, 1 cup, 250 mL	0	1.0	×	695	✓
Milk, Wheylike, 1 cup, 250 mL	0	3.0	×	350	✓
Milkshake, chocolate malted, 275 mL	0	12.0	×	1160	✓
Milky way bar, 1, 25g	0.5	4.0	××	455	××
Milkybar chew, 1, 22g	0	4.0	××	430	××
Milkybar, 1, 50g	0.5	17.5	××	1170	××
Milo dairy dessert, Bob the Builder, 100g	0	4.0	×	520	××
Milo dairy dessert, Monsters Inc, 100g	0	9.5	×	770	××
Milo dairy dessert, White chocolate, 100g	0	12.5	×	840	××
Milo, 3 tsp, 20g	0	2.0	×	350	×
Milo, malted, 4 tsp, 25g	0.5	2.5	×	440	×
Milo, Ready to drink, 600mL	0	21.5	×	2280	××
Mimosa, 130 mL	0	0		420	
Mince pie, home-made, 1	1.5	10.0	××	955	××
Mince pie, individual, double crust, 1	1.5	14.0	××	1185	××

Food	Fibre g	Fat g	Fat Rating	Energy kJ	Carb Rating
Mince tart, Bakers Delight, 1, 50g	1.0	7.5	××	870	××
Mince, savoury, canned, 220g	0.5	28.0	××	1665	×
Minced steak, 90% fat-free, raw, 100gt	0	10.0	×	685	
Minced steak, extra lean, 95% fat free, raw, 100g	0	5.0	×	540	
Minced steak, raw, 100g	0	11.0	×	740	
Mineral water & juice, 1 can, 370 mL	0	0		590	××
Mineral water, 1 glass, 250 mL	0	0		0	
Mineral water, flavoured, average, 1 can	0	0		650	××
Minestrone, large bowl	5.5	7.5	✓	665	✓✓
Mini wheats, 15, 30g	3.0	0		435	✓
Mint sauce, 1 tbsp	0	0		85	
Mint, fresh, 1 tbsp, 5g	0	0		10	
Mirin, 1 tbsp	0	0		190	
Miso soup, average bowl	0.5	3.0	✓	250	✓
Miso, soy bean paste, 1 tbsp, 20g	0	1.0	✓	170	✓
Mixed peel, 1 tbsp	1.0	0		100	××
Mixed vegetables, canned, ½ cup, 75g	2.0	0		110	✓
Mixed vegetables, frozen, 100g	6.0	0.5		140	✓
Molasses, 1 tbsp	0	0		300	×
Mortadella sausage, 50g	0.5	14.5	××	675	
Mountain bread, barley, 1 piece, 25g	1.0	0		195	✓
Mountain bread, corn, 1 piece, 25g	1.0	0.5		255	✓
Mountain bread, oat, 1 piece, 25g	1.0	0.5		240	✓
Mountain bread, rye, 1 piece, 25g	1.0	0		200	✓
Mountain bread, wheat, 1 piece, 25g	1.5	0.5		305	✓
Moussaka, average serve	2.0	26.0	×	1500	✓
Moussaka, Greek, average serve, 350g	3.0	33.5	×	2240	✓
Mud cake, average serve	4.0	82.0	××	4670	××
Muesli bar, apricot & coconut, average, 1, 31g	2.0	3.0	×	500	×
Muesli bar, apricot, 1, 32g	1.5	4.0	×	530	××

Food	Fibre g	Fat g	Fat Rating	Energy kJ	Carb Rating
Muesli bar, caramel, 1, 31g	1.5	3.0	××	515	××
Muesli bar, chewy apricot, 1, 31g	2.0	4.0	✓	510	××
Muesli bar, chewy choc chip, 1, 31g	1.5	4.0	××	540	×
Muesli bar, chewy forest fruits, 1, 31g	1.5	4.0	×	540	×
Muesli bar, chewy tropical, average, 1, 31g	2.0	3.0	×	500	×
Muesli bar, choc chip, average, 1, 31g	1.5	2.5	××	510	××
Muesli bar, choc chip, crunchy, 1, 30g	2.0	5.0	××	560	××
Muesli bar, choc malt, 1, 31g	1.5	4.5	×	560	××
Muesli bar, chocolate coated, average, 1, 33g	1.0	5.5	××	590	××
Muesli bar, crunchy apricot, average 1, 31g	2.0	4.0	×	570	×
Muesli bar, crunchy original, 1, 30g	2.5	6.5	×	580	×
Muesli bar, fruit & yoghurt, 1, 32g	1.5	5.5	×	570	×
Muesli bar, fruit topped, 1, 30g	2.0	2.0	×	455	×
Muesli bar, fruit, 1, 32g	1.5	4.5	×	495	×
Muesli bar, nut crumble, 1, 32g	1.5	6.0	×	600	×
Muesli bar, Weight Watchers, 1, 40g	1.5	0.5		480	×
Muesli bar, yoghurt top, 1, 31g	1.5	4.0	×	540	×
Muesli flakes, 1 cup, 40g	3.5	1.0	✓	560	✓
Muesli, Birchner, average serve, 230g	6.0	8.0	✓	1220	✓✓
Muesli, natural, ½ cup, 60g	6.0	4.5	✓✓	835	✓✓
Muesli, toasted, ½ cup, 60g	5.5	8.5	×	1030	✓
Muffin, cake type, 1, 150g	4.5	28.5	××	2320	××
Muffin, cake type, apple, 1	7.0	23.5	××	2000	××
Muffin, cake type, blueberry, 1	8.0	23.5	××	2045	××
Muffin, cake type, bran, 1	14.0	27.0	××	2310	×
Muffin, cake type, savoury, 1	3.5	22.5	××	1960	×
Muffin, cake type, wholemeal, 1	7.5	29.0	××	2645	×
Muffin, cake-type, 1 small, 60g	1.0	6.0	××	625	××
Muffin, cake-type, blueberry, 1 small, 60g	2.5	6.0	××	880	××
Muffin, English, 1, 67g	2.0	1.0	✓	700	✓
Muffin, fruit, 1, 67g	2.5	2.0	✓	700	✓

Food	Fibre g	Fat g	Fat Rating	Energy kJ	Carb Rating
Muffin, multigrain, 1, 67g	4.5	3.5	✓	700	✓✓
Muffin, Up, 1, 67g	2.5	3.0	✓✓	780	✓
Muffin, wholemeal, 1, 67g	3.5	2.0	✓	670	✓
Mulberries, ½ punnet, 100g	2.0	0		120	✓
Mullet, grilled, 150g	0	1.5	✓✓	615	
Multi-bran, ½ cup, 55g	11.5	7.0	✓✓	955	✓✓
Mung bean sprouts, ½ cup, 45g	1.5	0		80	
Mung beans, cooked, 1 cup, 200g	5.0	0.5		390	✓✓
Mung beans, dry, 100g	14.0	1.0	✓	1190	✓✓
Mushrooms, canned in sauce, ½ cup	1.5	1.5	✗	145	
Mushrooms, canned, whole, ½ cup	2.0	0		80	
Mushrooms, dried Chinese, 10g	1.5	0		120	✓
Mushrooms, dried, 6, 22g	2.5	0		270	✓
Mushrooms, enoki, 100g	2.5	0.5		140	✓
Mushrooms, fresh, 1 flat, 50g	1.5	0		50	
Mushrooms, fresh, button, 1 cup sliced, 100g	2.5	0		100	
Mushrooms, fresh, field, 1 large, 200g	6.0	0		530	✓
Mushrooms, marinated, 100g	2.0	1.5	✓	255	
Mushrooms, oyster, raw, 100g	3.0	0		35	
Mushrooms, portabella, raw, 100g	2.0	0		110	✓
Mushrooms, shiitake, cooked, ½ cup	2.0	0		160	✓
Mushrooms, shiitake, dried, 6 pieces, 25g	12.0	0		295	✓
Mushrooms, straw, canned, ½ cup	2.0	0		50	
Mushrooms, Swiss brown, 100g	1.5	0		90	
Mussels, fresh, 6	0	1.5	✓✓	330	
Mussels, smoked, 100g can, drained, 65g	0	8.5	✓✓	530	
Mustard & cress, ½ cup	1.0	0		15	
Mustard cabbage (gaai choi), 75g	1.5	0		50	
Mustard greens, 2 leaves	1.0	0		45	
Mustard powder, 1 tbsp, 10g	1.5	3.0	✓	220	
Mustard sauce, fast food portion, 1	0	4.0	✓	260	✗

Food	Fibre g	Fat g	Fat Rating	Energy kJ	Carb Rating
Mustard, Dijon, 2 tsp	0	1.0	✓	65	
Mustard, prepared, 2 tsp	0	0		30	
Mustard, wholegrain, 2 tsp	0.5	0.5		65	
Naan, 1 average, 80g	2.5	7.0	✓	960	✓
Naan, purchased, 1, 115g	3.5	6.0	✓	1260	✓
Nachos, average serving	12.0	60.0	×	3700	✓
Nashi pear, 1	2.5	0		185	✓✓
Neapolitan sauce, (for pasta), 1 cup	3.5	10.0	✓	540	✓
Nectarine, 1 average, 110g	2.5	0		155	✓✓
Neenish tart, 1, 45g	0.5	8.5	××	780	××
Nesquik ready to drink,, 250mL	0	6.0	×	785	××
Nesquik, powder, 2 tsp, 12g	0	0		205	××
Nik nax biscuits, 20, 20g	0	5.0	××	400	×
Noodles, cellophane, 50g	0	0		735	✓
Noodles, egg, cooked, 1 cup, 160g	1.5	0.5		425	✓✓
Noodles, egg, dry, 100g	2.5	1.5	×	1470	✓✓
Noodles, fried, 1 cup, 100g	1.0	11.5	××	640	✓
Noodles, Hokkien, Bamboo Pot, 150g	4.5	2.5	✓	1225	✓
Noodles, Hokkien, fresh, 150g	1.5	2.5	✓	1010	✓
Noodles, Kantong, 99% fat free, 150g	4.5	1.0	×	1010	✓
Noodles, mung bean, dry, 100g	0.5	0		1470	✓
Noodles, Pad Thai, 100g	1.0	2.0	×	560	✓
Noodles, rice fresh, 100g	1.0	0		850	✓
Noodles, rice, cooked, 1 cup, 175g	1.0	0.5		800	✓
Noodles, rice, dry, 100g	1.5	0.5		1525	✓
Noodles, soba, cooked, 1 cup, 115g	1.0	0.5		470	✓✓
Noodles, soba, dry, 100g	1.5	2.0	✓	1520	✓✓
Noodles, somen, cooked, 1 cup, 175g	3.0	0.5		965	✓✓
Noodles, somen, dry, 100g	4.5	1.0	✓	1490	✓✓
Noodles, Thai with vegetables, 250g serve	3.5	14.0	×	1660	✓
Noodles, Thai, Chiang mai, 200g	3.5	41.0	×	2400	✓

Food	Fibre g	Fat g	Fat Rating	Energy kJ	Carb Rating
Noodles, two minute, including flavour, 1 packet, 85g	0.5	15.0	××	1580	✓
Noodles, Udon, flavoured, 100g	2.0	0.5		460	✓✓
Noodles, wet, fresh, 100g	2.0	2.0	✓	480	✓✓
Noodles, wholemeal, dry, 100g	13.0	2.0	✓	1330	✓✓
Nori (seaweed), dried, 10 sheets, 5g	2.5	0		30	
Nut cutlets, 100g	3.0	22.0	✓	1205	✓✓
Nut roast, 100g	5.5	25.5	✓	1465	✓✓
Nutrigrain, 1 cup, 35g	1.0	0.5		560	×
Nuts, almonds, 50 g	4.5	28.0	✓✓	1240	
Nuts, Brazils, 50g	4.5	34.0	✓✓	1410	
Nuts, cashews, raw, 50g	3.0	24.5	✓✓	1195	
Nuts, cashews, roasted, 50g	3.0	25.5	✓✓	1310	
Nuts, coconut, fresh, 50g	4.0	14.5	××	560	
Nuts, hazelnuts, 50g	5.0	30.5	✓✓	1305	
Nuts, macadamia, 50g	3.0	38.0	✓✓	1510	
Nuts, mixed, 30g packet	2.5	16.0	✓✓	755	
Nuts, peanuts, 50g	4.0	26.0	✓✓	1285	
Nuts, pecans, 50g	4.0	36.0	✓✓	1455	
Nuts, pine nuts, 1 tbsp, 15g	1.0	10.5	✓✓	430	
Nuts, pistachios, 30g shelled	3.0	15.0	✓✓	695	
Nuts, walnut, ½ cup, 50g	3.0	35.0	✓✓	1425	
Oat Bran Bubbles, 1 cup, 30g	2.5	0		465	✓
Oat bran, crunchy, ½ cup, 50g	7.0	2.0	✓	720	✓
Oat bran, raw, ¼ cup, 35g	6.0	3.0	✓✓	520	✓✓
Oat Flakes, 1 cup, 50g	3.0	1.5	✓	765	✓
Oat milk, 250mL	0	4.5	✓✓	450	✓
Oats, rolled, cooked in water, 1 cup	2.0	2.5	✓✓	510	✓✓
Oats, rolled, cooked, ½ water, ½ milk, 1 cup	2.0	5.5	✓	630	✓✓
Oats, rolled, high fibre, raw, 1/2 cup, 60g	8.0	5.5	✓✓	900	✓✓
Oats, rolled, raw, ½ cup, 55g	4.0	4.5	✓✓	850	✓✓

Food	Fibre g	Fat g	Fat Rating	Energy kJ	Carb Rating
Octopus, 100g	0	0.5	✓	280	
Octopus, barbecued, 150 g	0	3.0	✓✓	1030	
Oil, any kind, 1 tbsp	0	20.0	✓	740	
Okra, cooked, 6 pods, 65g	3.0	0.5		80	✓
Okra, fried in oil, 3/4 cup	5.0	20.0	✓	840	✓
Okra, long (angled luffa), 75g	1.0	0		40	
Olive oil, any type, 1 tbsp	0	20.0	✓✓	740	
Olives, black, 6 medium, 40g	1.5	3.5	✓	135	
Olives, green, 6 medium, 50g	1.5	4.5	✓	170	
Olives, Kalamata, marinated, 20g	1.0	5.5g	✓	225	
Olives, Kalamata, mixed, brine, 20g	1.0	0.5g	✓	90	
Olives, Kalamata, plain, in oil, 20g	1.0	6.5g	✓	315	
Omelette, made from yolk-free egg	0	17.0	✓	930	
Omelette, plain or with herbs, 2 eggs	0	18.0	✗✗	860	
Omelette, Spanish potato, average wedge	2.0	18.0	✗✗	1150	
One minute oats, 1/2 cup, 45g	4.5	4.0	✓✓	690	✓✓
Onion, 1 medium	2.5	0		165	
Onion, brown, mature, raw, 1/2 cup, 80g	1.0	0		80	
Onion, rings, battered, deep-fried, 6 rings, 60g	0.5	16.0	✗✗	1020	
Onion, spring, 4, 50g	1.0	0		55	
Onion, white, mature, raw, 1/2 cup, 80g	1.0	0		90	
Onions, cocktail, pickled, 8, 40g	0.5	0		25	
Onions, dehydrated flakes, 1/4 cup, 20g	0.5	0		270	
Onions, fried, 1/2 cup, 100g	3.0	11.0	✗✗	685	
Onions, pickled, 2, 40g	0.5	0		40	
Orange & mango juice, 250 mL	0	0		565	✓
Orange flavour soft drink, 1 can, 370 mL	0	0		820	✗✗
Orange juice, freshly squeezed, 250 mL	0.5	0.5		470	✓✓
Orange juice, no sugar, prepared, 250 mL	0	0		355	✓✓
Orange juice, prepared, 250 mL	0	0		380	✓
Orange poppy seed cake, average serve	3.5	47.0	✗✗	2960	✗✗

Food	Fibre g	Fat g	Fat Rating	Energy kJ	Carb Rating
Orange, fresh, 1 medium, 180g	3.5	0		280	✓✓
Orange, fresh, 1 small, 125g	2.5	0		195	✓✓
Oregano, dried, 1 teaspoon, 2.5g	0.5	0.5		30	
Oregano, fresh, 1 tbsp chopped, 5g	0.5	0		15	
Oriental mix crackers, 25g	n/a	10.0	✗✗	555	✗
Osso buco, average serve	3.0	12.0	✗	1120	
Ostrich steak, cooked, 120g	0	1.5	✓	535	
OTs Fruity Bites, 1 cup, 35g	2.5	0.5		325	✓
Ovaltine light powder, 20g + 200 mL water	0	1.5	✓	335	✗
Ovaltine powder, 3 level teaspoons, 15g	0	0.5		200	✗
Ovaltine, 15g + 200 mL milk	0	8.0	✗	740	✗
Ovaltine, 15g + 200 mL skim milk	0	0.5		490	✗
Oxtail, stewed, 250g (weighed with bones)	0	13.0	✗	965	
Oysters Kilpatrick, 12	0	14.0	✗	1080	
Oysters, fresh, 6 medium	0	1.5	✓✓	180	
Oysters, smoked, 100g can, drained, 65g	0	8.0	✓	565	
Paddle pop, 1	0	3.5	✗	525	✗✗
Paella, average serve, 300g	2.0	16.5	✓	1790	✓
Pak choi (Chinese cabbage), cooked, ½ cup, 70g	2.0	0		40	
Pakora (Indian vegetable fritter), 1, 100g	6.0	10.0	✓	1040	✓
Palak paneer (Indian spinach & cheese), 150g	6.0	25.0	✗	1200	✓
Palm oil, 20g	0	20.0	✗✗	740	
Pancake with ice cream and topping	2.0	19.0	✗✗	2250	✗✗
Pancake with lemon and sugar	2.0	14.0	✗✗	1670	✗✗
Pancake, home-made, 1, 18cm, 60g	0.5	8.0	✗	565	✗
Paneer, kulcha (Indian fresh cheese), 50g	0	11.0	✗	780	
Panforte, small slice, 50g	3.0	11.0	✓	890	✗
Papaya green, 100g	1.5	0		115	✓
Papaya, 100g	1.0	0		160	✓
Pappadums, fried, 3 small	0.5	1.5	✓	155	✓

Food	Fibre g	Fat g	Fat Rating	Energy kJ	Carb Rating
Pappadums, grilled or microwaved, 3 small	0.5	0		70	✓
Pappadums, ready to eat, 3, 30g	0	0.5		430	✓
Paprika, dried powder, 1 tbsp, 10g	0	1.5	✓	120	
Paratha, ½ average, 60g	2.5	5.0	✓	555	✓
Parsley, ½ cup chopped, 30g	1.5	0.5		40	
Parsley, dried, 1 tbsp, 10g	4.5	0.5		75	
Parsley, Italian, ½ cup chopped, 30g	1.5	0		20	
Parsnip, sliced, steamed, ½ cup, 75g	2.0	0		155	✓
Partridge, roast, weighed with bone, 125g	0	7.5	✓	665	
Passionfruit, 1 average, 40g	3.0	0		40	✓
Pasta & sauce, beef satay, 1 serve, 125g	1.5	5.5	×	610	✓
Pasta & sauce, beef teriyaki 1 serve, 125g	1.5	5.5	×	630	✓
Pasta & sauce, beef/black bean 1 serve, 125g	1.5	5.5	×	655	✓
Pasta & sauce, chicken chow mein 1 serve, 125g	2.5	5.5	×	650	✓
Pasta & sauce, lemon chicken, 1 serve, 125g	1.5	5.5	×	645	✓
Pasta & sauce, satay prawn, 1 serve, 125g	1.5	6.0	×	630	✓
Pasta & sauce, spicy pork/plum sauce, 1 serve, 125g	1.5	5.5	×	625	✓
Pasta & sauce, sweet & sour pork, 1 serve, 125g	1.5	5.5	×	630	✓
Pasta and ham salad, 1 cup, 250g	6.5	20.0	×	1825	✓
Pasta arrabbiata, average serve	9.0	27.0	×	3060	✓✓
Pasta boscaiola, average serve	7.0	102.0	×	5570	✓✓
Pasta e fagioli, average serve	18.0	47.0	✓	3900	✓✓
Pasta pesto, average serve	10.0	44.0	✓	2800	✓✓
Pasta pesto, entrée serve	7.0	27.0	✓	2210	✓✓
Pasta primavera, average serve	14.0	34.0	×	3400	✓✓
Pasta sauce, Alfredo, restaurant, average serve	5.0	51.0	××	3445	×
Pasta sauce, basil & tomato, commercial, 1 cup	3.0	3.5	✓	625	✓
Pasta sauce, Latina carbonara, ½ cup	0	15.5	××	885	×
Pasta sauce, Latina creamy bacon/mushroom, ½ cup	n/a	17.0	××	840	×

Food	Fibre g	Fat g	Fat Rating	Energy kJ	Carb Rating
Pasta sauce, Latina hot Siciliana, ½ cup	n/a	3.0	✓	340	✓
Pasta sauce, Latina meat bolognaise, 1 cup	n/a	7.5	×	830	✓
Pasta sauce, Latina Mediterranean, ½ cup	2.5	5.0	✓	400	✓
Pasta sauce, Latina, cheese, ½ cup	0	18.0	××	975	✓
Pasta sauce, Leggo spicy tomato & bacon, ½ cup	n/a	6.0	×	440	✓
Pasta sauce, Roasted tomato, Paul Newman, 1 cup	5.0	6.0	✓	655	✓
Pasta sauce, Romano & garlic, commercial, 1 cup	n/a	9.5	✓	880	✓
Pasta sauce, tomato, commercial, 1 cup	5.5	2.0	✓	630	✓
Pasta sauce, tomato, home-made, average serve	7.5	5.0	✓	520	✓
Pasta, corn and parsley, dry, 100g	2.5	1.5	✓	1485	✓
Pasta, curly short, cooked, 1 cup, 145g	2.5	0.5		720	✓✓
Pasta, dry, 100g	5.0	1.0	✓	1430	✓✓
Pasta, egg, dry, 100g	2.5	1.5	✓	1470	✓✓
Pasta, fettucine, dry, 100g	5.0	2.0	✓	1450	✓✓
Pasta, fettucine, fresh, 150g	2.0	2.0	✓	1160	✓✓
Pasta, four cheeses, average serve	6.5	38.0	×	3390	✓✓
Pasta, fresh, 100g	3.5	1.5	✓	1100	✓✓
Pasta, less carbs, dry, 100g	17.5	2.0	✓	1230	✓✓
Pasta, mushroom sauce, average serve	8.0	7.0	✓	1750	✓✓
Pasta, Pan Sensations, chicken Alfredo, 330g	n/a	21.5	×	2090	✓
Pasta, Pan Sensations, with mushrooms, 330g	n/a	19.0	✓	2030	✓
Pasta, ricotta & spinach, 150g	4.0	7.0	×	1275	✓✓
Pasta, sauce, walnut cream, restaurant, average serve	8.0	79.0	×	4350	×
Pasta, spaghetti, cooked, 1 cup, 170g	3.0	0.5	✓	845	✓✓
Pasta, spaghetti, dry, 100g	5.0	2.0	✓	1455	✓✓
Pasta, spinach noodles, dry, 100g	4.5	1.5	✓	1490	✓✓
Pasta, wholemeal, cooked, 1 cup, 150g	8.5	1.0	✓	820	✓✓
Pasta, wholemeal, dry, 100g	13.0	2.0	✓	1330	✓✓
Pastizzi, spinach & ricotta pastries, 100g	n/a	9.5	×	900	×

Food	Fibre g	Fat g	Fat Rating	Energy kJ	Carb Rating
Pastry, cream horn, 1 65g	0.5	23.5	××	1170	××
Pastry, Danish, 100g	2.5	15.5	××	1290	××
Pastry, filo, 2 sheets, 34g	0.5	1.0	✓	440	✓
Pastry, flaky, average portion, 65g	1.0	26.0	××	1515	×
Pastry, puff, frozen, 1 sheet, 166g	2.0	37.0	××	2525	×
Pastry, puff, frozen, single crust, 75g	1.5	17.5	××	1170	×
Pastry, puff, home-made, 75g	1.5	21.0	××	1240	×
Pastry, shortcrust, frozen, raw, 100g	1.5	21.5	××	1375	×
Pastry, wholemeal, average portion, 65g	4.0	21.5	××	1350	✓
Pasty, 1, 165g	2.0	25.5	××	1815	✓
Pate, chicken liver, home-made, 100g	0	11.0	×	560	
Pate, liver, commercial, 50g	0	12.0	×	620	
Pavlova with cream & passionfruit, 1/8 30 cm	3.0	11.0	××	1325	××
Pawpaw, 100g	2.5	0		125	✓
Pawpaw, green, 100g	1.5	0		115	✓
Pea and ham soup, average bowl, 450g	8.5	4.0	×	1200	✓✓
Peach Melba, average serve	11.0	7.0	×	1500	✓
Peach, 1 large, 190g	2.5	0		250	✓✓
Peach, 1 medium, 140g	2.0	0		185	✓✓
Peach, 1 small, 100g	1.5	0		130	✓✓
Peach, dried, each half, 16g	1.5	0		160	✓✓
Peaches, canned in juice, sliced, 1 cup, 250g	3.5	0		425	✓✓
Peaches, canned syrup, drained, 2 halves	1.0	0		170	✓
Peaches, canned syrup, sliced, 1 cup, 250g	3.5	0		550	✓
Peaches, canned water, sliced, 1 cup, 250g	3.5	0		260	✓✓
Peaches, canned, pie pack, ½ cup, 120g	1.5	0		125	✓✓
Peaches, canned, snack pack in jelly, 140g	2.0	0		400	✓
Peaches, canned, snack pack, 140g	2.0	0		320	✓✓
Peaches, canned, syrup, 2 halves	2.0	0		285	✓
Peanut brittle, 50g	0	6.5	×	900	××
Peanut butter, 1 tbsp, 25g	2.5	13.0	✓	620	

Food	Fibre g	Fat g	Fat Rating	Energy kJ	Carb Rating
Peanut oil, 1 tbsp	0	20.0	✓	740	
Peanut sauce, ¼ cup	3.5	24.0	××	1100	
Peanuts, 50g	4.0	26.0	✓	1285	
Pear juice (in canned fruit), ½ cup	0	0		230	×
Pear, canned in syrup, 2 halves with syrup	3.0	0		460	✓
Pear, canned in syrup, drained, 2 halves	3.0	0		300	✓
Pear, canned in water, 2 halves	2.5	0		250	✓✓
Pear, canned, snack pack, 140g	2.5	0		345	✓✓
Pear, dried, each half, 20g	2.0	0		200	✓✓
Pear, fresh, Beurre bosc, 1 medium, 220g	5.5	0		520	✓✓
Pear, fresh, Packham, 1 medium, 160g	4.0	0		350	✓✓
Pear, fresh, William, 1 medium, 175g	4.0	0		345	✓✓
Peas, dried, 100g	15.0	2.5	✓	1290	✓✓
Peas, dried, cooked, 1 cup, 135g	7.0	1.0	✓	630	✓✓
Peas, fresh, green, raw, 100g	5.5	0.5		250	✓✓
Peas, green with edible pods, 100g	4.0	0		135	✓
Peas, green, cooked, ½ cup, 80g	5.0	0.5		160	✓✓
Peas, green, frozen, cooked, ½ cup, 80g	4.5	0.5		170	✓✓
Peas, mushy, canned, 100g	8.0	0.5		335	✓✓
Peas, snow, 50g	2.0	0		80	✓
Peas, split, green/yellow, cooked, 1 cup, 170g	6.5	0.5		410	✓✓
Peas, split, green/yellow, dry, 100g	10.0	2.0	✓	1240	✓✓
Peas, split, red, cooked, 1 cup, 180g	7.0	0.5		455	✓✓
Peas, split, red, dry, ½ cup, 95g	9.5	2.0	✓	1180	✓✓
Peas, sugar-snap, 100g	4.0	0		145	✓
Pecan nuts, 50g	4.0	36.0	✓	1455	
Pecan pie, 1/8 23 cm pie	2.5	33.0	×	2175	××
Pepino, 1 medium, 120g	1.5	0		110	✓
Pepitas, (pumpkin seeds), ½ cup, 35g	12.5	7.0	✓	650	✓✓
Pepper steak, 200g	0	36.0	×	2250	

Food	Fibre g	Fat g	Fat Rating	Energy kJ	Carb Rating
Pepper, (capsicum) yellow, raw, ½ medium, 110g	2.0	0		100	
Pepper, (capsicum), green, raw, ½ medium, 90g	1.5	0		60	
Pepper, (capsicum), red, raw, ½ medium, 110g	1.5	0		115	
Pepper, banana chilli, each, 80g	1.0	0		45	
Pepper, cayenne, ¼ teaspoon, 1g	0	0		15	
Pepper, chilli, long thin, 80g	2.0	0		80	
Pepper, chilli, red, each, 20g	0.5	0		25	
Pepper, chilli, small green, each, 20g	0.5	0		15	
Peppermint lifesavers, 1 packet, 20g	0	0		335	
Peppermints, 4, 10g	0	0		165	
Pepperoni, 50g	0	18.0	××	885	
Peppers, roasted, drained, 1/4 cup	0.5	0		55	
Persimmon, 1 medium, 120g	3.0	0		335	
Pesto, ¼ cup	1.0	45.0	✓	1740	
Pharo crisps, average 50g	2.5	3.0	✓	850	✓
Pheasant, roast, weighed with bone, 125g	0	7.5	×	700	
Pie, pecan, 1/8 23 cm pie	2.5	33.0	××	2175	××
Pigeon peas, dried, 100g	16.5	2.0	✓	1350	✓✓
Pigeon peas, dried, cooked, ½ cup, 90g	6.0	0.5		450	✓✓
Pigeon, breast, roast, 100g	0	13.0	✓	960	
Pigeon, roast, weighed with bone, 125g	0	7.0	✓	525	
Pigs trotters, cooked, 1	0	15.5	×	700	
Pikelets, 1 7.5cm	0	2.5	×	210	✓
Pilaf, home-made, average serve	1.5	3.5	✓	890	✓
Pilchards in tomato sauce, canned, 100g	0	5.5	✓✓	530	
Pilchards, floured & fried, 150g	0	10.0	✓✓	740	
Pine nuts, 1 tbsp, 15g	1.0	10.5	✓✓	430	
Pineapple juice, unsweetened, 250 mL	0	0		490	✓
Pineapple upside down cake, average serve	2.0	20.0	××	1550	××

Food	Fibre g	Fat g	Fat Rating	Energy kJ	Carb Rating
Pineapple, canned in juice, drained, 1 cup, 215g	3.5	0		400	✓
Pineapple, canned in syrup, 1 slice, 55g	0.5	0		195	✓
Pineapple, canned in syrup, drained, 1 slice, 35g	0.5	0		125	✓
Pineapple, crushed, canned in juice, 1 cup, 250g	4.0	0		465	✓
Pineapple, fresh, 1 slice, 120g	2.5	0		190	✓
Pissaladiere (onion tart), ¼ 20 cm pie	6.0	26.0	✗✗	1995	✓
Pistachio nuts, 30g shelled	3.0	15.0	✓✓	695	
Pistachio nuts, weighed in shells, 100g	6.0	30.5	✓✓	1370	
Pita bread, 1 medium, 90g	3.5	1.0	✓	1000	✓
Pita crisps, 50g	1.5	8.5	✗	910	✓
Pizza base, home-made, ¼ 30cm pizza	5.0	6.0	✓	1400	✓
Pizza roll, 1, 100g	3.0	11.0	✗	1245	✓
Pizza slice supreme, Bakers Delight, 200g	5.0	20.5	✗	1965	✓
Pizza slice, vegetarian, Bakers Delight, 165g	4.5	16.5	✗	1715	✓
Pizza thin 'n crispy, cheese, ¼, 120g	2.5	14.0	✗	1380	✓
Pizza thin 'n crispy, Hawaiian, ¼, 150g	3.0	14.5	✗	1540	✓
Pizza thin 'n crispy, super supreme, ¼, 175g	3.5	21.0	✗	1820	✓
Pizza thin 'n crispy, supreme, ¼, 170g	3.0	19.0	✗	1785	✓
Pizza, boboli base, 1, 112g	3.0	5.0	✓	1245	✓
Pizza, ham & mushroom, home-made, 12 cm diam	5.0	22.0	✗	2390	✓
Pizza, home-made, vegetarian, ¼ 30cm pizza	10.0	16.0	✓	2035	✓
Pizza, Neapolitan, home-made, 12 cm diam.	5.0	17.0	✗	2165	✓
Pizza, pan Hawaiian, ¼,185g	4.0	16.0	✗	1840	✓
Pizza, pan super supreme, ¼, 215g	4.5	22.5	✗	2140	✓
Pizza, pan supreme, ¼, 200g	4.0	24.5	✗	2150	✓
Pizza, pan, cheese, ¼, 160g	3.5	16.0	✗	1665	✓
Plantain, fresh, 1 medium, 200g with skin	4.5	0.5		660	✓✓
Plum pudding, rich, 1/10 pudding	7.0	34.0	✗✗	3640	✗

Food	Fibre g	Fat g	Fat Rating	Energy kJ	Carb Rating
Plum, blood, 2 average, 200g	4.5	0		310	✓✓
Plum, canned in syrup, 1 cup, 255g	4.5	0		920	✓
Plum, canned in syrup, drained, 1 cup, 220g	4.5	0		810	✓
Plum, Damson variety, 2 average, 130g	4.5	0		190	✓✓
Plum, yellow flesh, 2 average, 180g	3.5	0		230	✓✓
Polenta, average serve	2.0	1.5	✓	865	✓✓
Polenta, dry corn meal, 100g	3.0	2.0	✓	1380	✓✓
Polony sausage, 50g	0	10.5	✗✗	585	
Pomegranate, 1 medium, 300g with skin	9.0	0		395	✓
Pomelo, 1 medium, 500g with skin	1.5	0		390	✓✓
Pop tarts, Apple Cinnamon, 1, 50g	1.0	5.5	✓	825	✗✗
Pop tarts, Berry, 1, 50g	1.0	5.5	✓	815	✗✗
Pop tarts, Double Choc, 1, 50g	1.0	5.0	✓	825	✗✗
Popcorn, candied, 1 cup, 20g	1.5	2.0	✗	330	✗
Popcorn, home cooked, 1 cup, 10g	1.0	2.0	✓	175	✓
Popcorn, plain, commercial, 1 cup, 10g	1.0	2.5	✓	195	✓
Poppy seeds, 1 cup, 140g	14.0	61.5	✓	3120	
Poppy seeds, 1 tbsp,	1.0	4.5	✓	225	
Pork bun, Chinese, 1	2.0	12.0	✗	1300	✓
Pork pie, 1, 175g	1.5	47.0	✗✗	2735	✗
Pork rind snack food, (crackling), 30g	0	8.5	✗✗	610	
Pork sausage, extra lean, 100g	0	8.0	✗	665	
Pork sausage, grilled, 1, 80g	1.0	17.5	✗	950	
Pork, barbecued Chinese, 100g	0	15.0	✗	995	
Pork, belly, grilled, 100g	0	35.0	✗	1645	
Pork, butterfly steak, trimmed, grilled, 100g	0	4.5	✗	675	
Pork, chop suey, average serve, 150g	2.5	13.0	✗	1010	✓
Pork, leg steak, grilled, lean & fat, 100g	0	6.0	✗	720	
Pork, leg steak, grilled, lean only, 95g	0	5.5	✗	620	
Pork, loin chop, baked, lean & fat, 1, 100g	0	30.0	✗	1520	
Pork, loin chop, baked, lean only, 1, 70g	0	3.5	✗	500	

Food	Fibre g	Fat g	Fat Rating	Energy kJ	Carb Rating
Pork, medallion steak, trimmed, grilled, 100g	0	6.5	×	785	
Pork, plum sauce, average serve, 150g	0	26.0	×	1535	
Pork, roast leg, lean & fat, 2 slices, 90g	0	24.0	×	1275	
Pork, roast leg, lean only, 2 slices, 70g	0	3.0	×	500	
Pork, shoulder chop, 1, baked, lean & fat, 145g	0	41.0	×	2070	
Pork, shoulder chop, 1, baked, lean only, 100g	0	8.0	×	760	
Pork, spare ribs, black bean sauce, 200g	2.0	29.0	×	1670	✓
Pork, sweet & sour, home-made, average serve	0.5	52.0	×	2700	×
Pork, sweet & sour, restaurant, average serve, 250g	0.5	23.5	××	1925	×
Porridge, see oats					
Port, 1 glass, 60 mL	0	0		400	
Potato baked (olive oil spray, 1 medium, 150g	4.5	0.5		870	✓
Potato flakes, raw, 25g	3.5	0		340	✓
Potato wedges, 6, 200g	3.0	20.0	××	1965	✓
Potato, 1 medium cooked, 150g	2.0	0		390	✓
Potato, 1 small, cooked, skin on, 100g	1.5	0		275	✓
Potato, 1 small, peeled, cooked, 100g	1.0	0		275	✓
Potato, and leek soup, average bowl, 250g	1.5	8.5	×	555	✓
Potato, baked in jacket, 200g	2.5	0		455	✓
Potato, boiled or steamed, 1, 150g	2.5	0.5		475	✓
Potato, cakes, 1, 50g	1.0	8.0	×	500	✓
Potato, canned, peeled, 6 small, 170g	2.5	0		400	✓
Potato, chips, fine cut, commercial, fried, 100g	3.5	21.5	××	1525	✓
Potato, chips, frozen oven-cook, 100g	4.5	8.0	×	1150	✓
Potato, chips, frozen oven-cook, super fries, 100g	4.5	7.0	×	700	✓
Potato, chips, home-fried in oil, drained, 100g	3.5	8.5	✓	795	✓
Potato, chips, hot, commercial, average serve, 150g	5.5	21.0	××	1545	✓
Potato, chips, thick cut, home-fried in oil, 100g	3.5	10.0	✓	985	✓
Potato, crisps, 50g packet	6.0	16.0	××	1050	×

Food	Fibre g	Fat g	Fat Rating	Energy kJ	Carb Rating
Potato, crisps, flavoured, 50g packet	6.0	16.5	××	1085	×
Potato, crisps, Lites, 50g packet	6.0	16.5	××	1065	×
Potato, crisps, Pringles, cheese, ¼ packet, 43g	5.0	16.0	××	1025	×
Potato, crisps, Pringles, corn, ¼ packet, 43g	5.0	10.5	××	900	×
Potato, crisps, Pringles, light, ¼ packet, 43g	5.0	11.0	××	920	×
Potato, flakes, mashed with milk, ½ cup, 100g	2.5	1.0	×	325	✓
Potato, flour, 100g	2.0	0.5		1380	✓
Potato, gems, 10, 100g	5.5	13.0	××	1030	✓
Potato, gnocchi, home-made, av serve	6.5	3.5	×	2045	✓
Potato, hash browns, commercial, 56g	1.0	12.0	××	730	✓
Potato, hash browns, home-made, ½ cup, 80g	1.0	11.0	××	700	✓
Potato, mashed, restaurant, average serve	2.5	28.0	××	1540	✓
Potato, mashed, with butter, 1 cup, 200g	2.5	7.0	×	775	✓
Potato, mashed, without butter, 1 cup, 200g	2.5	1.5	×	570	✓
Potato, new, 6 small, 165g	3.0	0		435	✓
Potato, omelette, Spanish, average wedge	2.0	18.0	×	1150	✓
Potato, pancakes, each, 200g	2.5	9.5	×	850	✓
Potato, roasted in oil, 100g piece	2.5	4.5	✓	630	✓
Potato, roesti, average serve	5.0	14.0	×	1260	✓
Potato, salad, canned, average serve, 100g	1.0	7.0	✓	500	×
Potato, salad, commercial, average serve, 100g	1.0	4.5	✓	450	✓
Potato, salad, home-made, vinaigrette dressing,	2.5	18.0	✓	1050	✓
Potato, salad, home-made, with mayonnaise, ½ cup	1.0	18.0	✓	940	✓
Potato, scallop, deep fried, each 100g	1.5	21.5	××	1350	✓
Potato, shoestring fries, 150g	3.5	11.0	××	1180	×
Potato, straws, 50g packet	6.0	14.5	××	1045	×
Potato, straws, flavoured, 50g packet	6.0	15.5	××	1075	×
Powerbar, Protein Plus78g	3.0	5.0	×	1260	××
Prawn & coconut milk curry, average serve	1.0	21.0	×	1290	
Prawn chow mein, average serve, 150g	1.0	16.5	×	910	✓

Food	Fibre g	Fat g	Fat Rating	Energy kJ	Carb Rating
Prawn cocktail, average serve, 125g	0	9.0	×	635	
Prawn crisps, 25g	0.5	8.5	×	540	×
Prawn cutlets, 3, 75g	0	11.0	✓	825	×
Prawn omelette, average 150g	0	23.0	✓	1150	
Prawns, curried with rice, average serve, 250g	2.0	14.0	✓	1125	✓
Prawns, curried, average serve	2.0	14.0	✓	845	
Prawns, king, 3	0	0.5	✓✓	240	
Prawns, school, cooked, weighed in shells, 100g	0	1.0	✓✓	420	
Prawns, sweet & sour, average serve, 140g	1.0	5.5	✓	690	×
Premium crackers, 6, 22g	0.5	4.0	×	425	×
Pretzels, 30g	1.0	1.0	×	470	×
Prickly pear, 1 medium, 90g	7.0	0		150	✓
Pro-Activ spread, 1 tbsp	0	13.0	✓	480	
Profiteroles, chocolate, 1, 5cm x 75 cm	0.5	14.0	××	835	××
Protein powders, average, 100g	0	1.0	×	1490	✓
Prune juice, 250 mL	2.0	0		660	✓
Prunes, 6 medium	4.5	0		465	✓
Prunes, canned, ½ cup, 140g	8.0	0		640	✓
Prunes, pitted, 50g	6.5	0		530	✓
Pudding, bread, average serve	3.0	9.5	×	1365	×
Pudding, chocolate self-saucing, average. Serve	1.5	10.0	×	1700	×
Pudding, Christmas, rich, 1/10 pudding	7.0	34.0	××	3640	×
Pudding, lemon delicious, average serve	0.5	11.0	××	995	××
Pudding, plum, home-made, 1/10 pudding	5.5	19.5	××	2560	×
Pudding, sago, home-made, average serve	0	9.0	×	850	×
Pudding, self-saucing, canned, 100g	1.0	7.0	×	970	××
Pudding, steamed, average serve. 100g	1.0	16.0	××	1440	××
Puff pastry, frozen, 75g	1.5	17.5	××	1170	×
Puff pastry, home-made, 75g	1.5	21.0	××	1240	×
Puffed wheat, 1 cup, 30g	2.0	0.5		465	✓

Food	Fibre g	Fat g	Fat Rating	Energy kJ	Carb Rating
Pumpkin flowers, 6, 12g	0	0		10	
Pumpkin flowers, deep fried in light batter, 6	0.5	15.0	×	750	×
Pumpkin pie, 1/8 23 cm pie	2.0	24.5	××	1830	××
Pumpkin scones, each, 40g	1.0	3.5	×	420	✓
Pumpkin seeds (pepitas), 25g	3.5	11.0	✓✓	590	
Pumpkin soup, home-made,1 bowl	2.0	10.0	×	690	✓
Pumpkin, butternut, average piece, cooked, 85g	1.5	0.5		165	✓
Pumpkin, nuggett, average piece, cooked, 75g	0.5	0		95	✓
Pumpkin, Queensland blue, cooked, 85g	1.5	0		175	✓
Pumpkin, roast, average piece, 75g	1.0	4.0	×	280	✓
Puri (Indian bread), 1, 45g	1.0	5.0	×	560	✓
Purslane, 1 cup, 45g	0.5	0		30	
Quail, flesh and skin, 1 bird	0	13.0	✓	875	
Quail, flesh, lean only, raw, 1 bird	0	4.0	✓	515	
Quark, 100g	0	0		305	
Quiche Lorraine, average serve	1.5	44.0	××	2400	×
Quiche Lorraine, purchased, 1 serve, 240g	1.5	35.0	××	2425	×
Quiche, frozen, 1/4, 125g	1.0	27.5	××	1640	×
Quiche, frozen, light, 1/4, 150g	1.0	14.5	××	1000	×
Quiche, mushroom, purchased, 1/4, 110g	2.0	17.0	××	1170	×
Quiche, spinach, purchased, 1/4, 110g	3.0	17.0	××	1330	×
Quince paste, 50g	0	0		510	×
Quince, 1/2 medium, 110g cooked in syrup	8.0	0		380	✓
Quince, stewed with sugar, 1	12.0	0.5		880	×
Quorn, 100g	5.0	3.5	✓	360	
Rabbit casserole, average serve	1.5	8.0	✓	1280	
Rabbit in mustard cream sauce, average serve	0	39.0	×	2650	
Rabbit, meat only, cooked, 100g	0	4.0	✓	380	
Radicchio, 1 cup	1.0	0		20	
Radish leaves, 1 cup	1.5	0		55	
Radish, red skin, 2 medium, 40g	0.5	0		20	

Food	Fibre g	Fat g	Fat Rating	Energy kJ	Carb Rating
Radish, white, 1 cup sliced, 90g	1.5	0.5		65	
Rainbow trout. 100g	0	3.0	✓	525	
Raisin bread, 1 slice, 30g	1.0	0.5		325	
Raisins, 30g	1.5	0		365	
Raspberries, 1/2 punnet, 100g	6.5	0		110	✓
Raspberries, canned in syrup, 1/2 cup	8.0	0		475	✓
Raspberries, frozen, 100g	9.5	0		155	✓
Ratatouille, average serve	5.0	7.0	✓	440	✓
Ravioli, 96% fat free, canned, 220g	3.5	8.5	×	925	✓
Ravioli, canned, 1/2 can, 220g	3.5	11.0	××	1200	✓
Ravioli, home-made, 180g	2.5	24.0	×	1920	✓✓
Ravioli, ready to cook, serve recommended, 125g	4.0	17.0	✓	1490	✓✓
Ready Wheats, 20, 30g	3.0	1.0	✓	460	✓
Redcurrant jelly, 1 tbsp	0	0		205	××
Re-fried beans, canned, 1 cup	9.5	1.5	✓	680	✓✓
Re-fried beans, restaurant, 1 cup	16.5	21.0	✓	1575	✓✓
Relish, home-made tomato, 1 tbsp	0.5	0		80	
Rhubarb, raw, 100g	3.0	0		75	
Rhubarb, stewed with sugar, 1/2 cup	6.0	0		475	×
Rib eye, grilled, lean & fat, 1 small steak, 130g	0	22.0	××	1260	
Rib eye, grilled, lean only, 1 small steak, 110g	0	6.0	×	815	
Ribena, undiluted, 25 mL	0	0		245	
Rice and corn pasta, dry, 100g	2.5	1.5	✓	1550	✓
Rice beverage, 250 mL	0	2.0	✓	510	✓
Rice bran, crunchy, 1/2 cup, 55g	14.0	11.0	✓	975	✓
Rice bubbles, 1 cup, 30g	0.5	0		480	×
Rice cakes, plain, 2	0.5	0.5		355	×
Rice cracker snacks, 1 cup, 60g	0.5	0.5		960	×
Rice cracker snacks, 1 packet, 150g	0.5	0.5		2310	×
Rice crackers, plain, 6, 10g	0	0.5		175	×

Food	Fibre g	Fat g	Fat Rating	Energy kJ	Carb Rating
Rice Creme, Attiki, 100g	0	3.0	×	495	✓
Rice Crispies, 1 cup, 30g	0	0.5		460	×
Rice Doongara, raw, 100g	0.5	0.5		1470	✓✓
Rice dream milk, 1 cup, 250 mL	0	4.5	✓	525	✓
Rice Flakes with psyllium, 50g	4.0	1.0	✓	750	✓✓
Rice flour, 1 tbsp, 12g	0	0		180	✓
Rice meals, Chinese, 1/2 packet cooked	n/a	3.0	×	1125	
Rice meals, Creole, 1/2 packet cooked	n/a	3.5	×	1170	
Rice meals, Hawaiian, 1/2 packet cooked	n/a	5.0	×	1200	
Rice meals, Indian, 1/2 packet cooked	n/a	3.5	×	1080	
Rice meals, satay rice, 1/2 packet cooked	n/a	9.0	×	1480	
Rice milk, 1 cup, 250 mL	0	3.0	✓	525	✓
Rice nibbles, 1 packet, 100g	0.5	23.0	××	2100	××
Rice noodles, see noodles					
Rice paper wrap, 1, 10g	0	0		140	✓
Rice pudding, canned, 150g	0.5	4.0	×	560	×
Rice pudding, canned, banana, 150g	2.0	9.5	×	690	×
Rice pudding, canned, chocolate, 150g	2.0	4.5	×	590	×
Rice pudding, canned, vanilla, 150g	2.0	2.5	×	510	×
Rice pudding, creamy, average serve, 160g	0	8.0	×	680	×
Rice white & wild rice blend, 100g	1.5	1.0	✓	1480	✓
Rice, Basmati, raw, 100g	2.5	0.5		1500	✓✓
Rice, brown, cooked, 1 cup, 160g	3.0	1.5	✓	1000	✓
Rice, brown, raw, 100g	4.0	2.5	✓	1530	✓
Rice, fried, average serve	2.0	13.5	××	1490	✓
Rice, glutinous, 100g	0.5	1.5	✓	1500	✓
Rice, sungold, cooked, 1 cup, 160g	1.5	0.5		830	✓
Rice, sungold, raw, 100g	3.0	1.0	✓	1510	✓
Rice, white, cooked, 1 cup, 175g	1.5	0.5		915	✓
Rice, white, raw, 100g	2.0	0.5		1470	✓
Rice, wild, 100g	6.0	1.0	✓	1495	✓

Food	Fibre g	Fat g	Fat Rating	Energy kJ	Carb Rating
Ricotta, see under cheese					
Ris O'Mais, Orgran, dry, 100g	2.5	0.5		1380	✓
Risotto, average serve, 250g	1.5	10.5	✓	1220	✓
Rissoles, 2, 340g	3.5	31.0	×	2780	×
Rissoles, beef, cheese & honey, 2, 150g	0	23.0	×	1190	×
Rissoles, lamb, cheese & honey, 2, 150g	0	23.0	×	1390	×
Rissoles, pork, cheese & honey, 2, 150g	0	24.0	×	1390	×
Roast beef, topside, 2 slices, lean & fat, 90g	0	9.0	×	720	
Roast beef, topside, 2 slices, lean only, 80g	0	4.0	×	570	
Roasted capsicum, drained, 1/2 cup	1.5	1.5	✓	185	
Roasted hot peppers, drained, 1/4 cup	0.5	0		55	
Rocket, 1 cup, 30g	1.0	0		45	
Rockmelon, 1 cup cubed, 150g	1.5	0		135	✓
Rockmelon, 1/4 medium, peeled, 175g	2.0	0		160	
Rockmelon, wedge, 250g	2.5	0		230	
Roe, fish, black 10g	0	0.5		40	
Roe, fish, red 10g	0	1.0		65	
Roesti, average serve	5.0	14.0	××	1260	✓
Rogan josh (lamb curry), average serve	5.0	36.0	×	2200	✓
Roll up, fruit, 1, 15g	0	0.5		240	××
Rolled oat, see oats					
Rose apple, (wax jambu) 1 medium, 35g	0.5	0		35	✓
Rosehip syrup, undiluted, 25 mL	0	0		250	×
Rosellas, 1 cup, 60g	n/a	0		125	✓
Rosemary, dried, 1 teaspoon, 2.5g	0	0.5		35	
Rosemary, fresh, 1 tbsp chopped, 5g	0.5	0		20	
Roti wrap, 1, 45g	1.5	4.0	✓	660	✓
Roti, average serve, 80g	2.0	5.0	✓	1100	✓
Round steak, 100g raw, lean & fat	0	12.0	×	800	
Round steak, 100g raw, lean only	0	4.5	×	555	
Round steak, grilled, 150g, lean & fat	0	15.0	×	1275	

Food	Fibre g	Fat g	Fat Rating	Energy kJ	Carb Rating
Round steak, grilled, lean only, 145g	0	9.0	×	1070	
Rum balls, home-made, each, 15g	0.5	4.0	××	265	××
Rum, 1 nip, 30 mL	0	0		265	
Rump centre steak, grilled, 130g	0	6.5	×	805	
Rump steak eye, grilled, 130g	0	5.5	×	780	
Rump steak, grilled, lean & fat, 1 steak, 200g	0	33.5	×	2260	
Rump steak, grilled, lean only, 1 steak, 150g	0	10.0	×	1200	
Rusks, baby, each, 8g	0	0.5		120	×
Rutabaga (swede), 1/2 cup pieces, cooked, 85g	2.0	0		40	✓
Rye flour, 1 cup	16.0	3.0	✓	2000	✓
Rye, wholegrain, ½ cup	9.5	1.5	✓	1140	✓✓
Ryvita, 2 slices	2.5	2.0	✓	340	✓
Safflower oil, 1 tbsp	0	20.0	✓	740	
Safflower seed kernels, 1 tbsp, 10g	0.5	4.0	✓✓	215	
Saffron, 1/4 teaspoon, 1g	0	0		15	
Sage, dried, 1 teaspoon, 2.5g	0	0.5		35	
Sago pudding, home-made, average serve	0	9.0	×	850	×
Salad cream, 1 tbsp	0	6.0	×	290	
Salad cream, light, 1 tbsp	0	4.0	×	210	
Salad with soba noodles, entree size	4.0	42.0	✓	1940	✓✓
Salad, Caesar, average serve, 280g	4.5	30.0	×	1850	
Salad, Waldorf, average serve, 140g	3.0	18.0	✓	1030	✓
Salami, Danish, 50g	0	20.0	×	930	
Salami, fat-reduced, 50g	0	9.0	×	515	
Salami, Hans reduced fat, 50g	0	10.0	×	665	
Salami, Hungarian, 50g	0	19.0	×	890	
Salami, Mettwurst, 50g	0	19.0	×	895	
Salami, Milano, 50g	0	18.5	×	890	
Salami, pepperoni, 50g	0	18.0	×	885	
Salami, Polish, 50g	0.5	9.0	×	500	
Salmon, Atlantic, grilled, 150g	0	4.0	✓✓	765	

Food	Fibre g	Fat g	Fat Rating	Energy kJ	Carb Rating
Salmon, Australian, canned, 100g (drained 88g)	0	1.0	✓✓	400	
Salmon, canned, pink, 100g (drained 88g)	0	6.0	✓	545	
Salmon, canned, red, 100g (drained 88g)	0	10.5	✓✓	720	
Salmon, canned, skinless, 100g	0	4.0	✓✓	535	
Salmon, mousse, average serve, 125g	0	15.0	××	885	×
Salmon, patty mix, 100g	0	7.5	✓	850	×
Salmon, smoked pate, 1 serve, 40g	0	9.0	×	470	
Salmon, smoked, 50g	0	2.5	✓✓	280	
Salsa	1.0	0		75	
Salsify, sliced, cooked, 1/2 cup, 70g	1.5	0		75	
Saltines, 3, 22g	0.5	4.5	×	420	×
Samosa, meat, 1, 80g	1.5	44.0	××	1960	×
Samosa, small, 2, 80g	1.0	22.0	××	1050	×
Samosa, vegetable, 1 average, 145g	3.5	18.5	××	1610	×
San bran, 1/2 cup, 45g	15.0	4.0	✓	480	✓
Sandwich fillings, avocado and salad	1.5	11.0	✓	460	
Sandwich fillings, cheese	0	10.0	×	485	
Sandwich fillings, chicken	0	5.0	✓	415	
Sandwich fillings, corned beef, lean	0	1.5	×	205	
Sandwich fillings, corned beef, lean and fat	0	4.5	×	315	
Sandwich fillings, cream cheese	0	13.0	××	570	
Sandwich fillings, egg	0	5.0	✓	285	
Sandwich fillings, egg and mayonnaise	0	11.0	✓	580	
Sandwich fillings, ham	0	3.5	×	265	
Sandwich fillings, lentil patty	3.0	1.0	✓	450	✓✓
Sandwich fillings, peanut butter	2.5	13.0	✓	620	
Sandwich fillings, prawns in mayonnaise	0	6.5	✓	490	
Sandwich fillings, roast beef	0	2.5	×	320	
Sandwich fillings, salad	1.0	0.0		35	
Sandwich fillings, smoked salmon	0	2.0	✓✓	230	

Food	Fibre g	Fat g	Fat Rating	Energy kJ	Carb Rating
Sandwich fillings, smoked salmon, cream cheese, capers	0	15.0	✓	825	
Sandwich fillings, sun-dried tomato, eggplant, zucchini, roasted capsicum	1.5	10.0	✓	440	
Sandwich fillings, tuna in mayonnaise	0	7.5	✓✓	530	
Sandwich, 2 slices white bread, no spread	1.5	1.5	✓	625	✓
Sandwich, 2 slices white bread/margarine	1.5	13.0	✓	1035	✓
Sandwich, 2 slices w'meal or multigrain, no spread	4.0	1.5	✓	565	✓✓
Sandwich, 2 slices w'meal or multigrain/margarine	4.0	13.0	✓	980	✓✓
Sandwich, focaccia, bread only 80g	2.0	12.0	✓	1100	✓
Sandwich, Turkish bread, bread only, 80g	2.0	2.0	✓	725	✓
Sao biscuits, 2, 18g	0.5	3.0	×	330	×
Sapodilla, 100g	8.0	1.0	✓	290	✓
Sapote, 100g	2.5	0.5		560	✓
Sardines, canned in tomato sauce, 100g	0	11.5	✓✓	740	
Sardines, grilled, 4	0	5.0	✓✓	400	
Sardines, in brine or water, 100g can	0	8.0	✓✓	600	
Sardines, in oil, 100g can, (drained 80g)	0	12.5	✓✓	760	
Sarsparilla soft drink, 1 can, 370 mL	0	0		730	××
Satay rice, made as directed, 1 cup	1.0	5.0	×	1610	✓
Satay sauce, commercial, ½ cup	0	14.0	×	1215	×
Satay sauce, home-made, 1/2 cup	4.0	29.0	×	1420	
Satsumas (mandarins), 1 average, 50g	1.5	0		130	✓
Sauce, aioli, 1 tbsp, 20g	0	16.0	✓	610	
Sauce, Alfredo, average serve	0	45.0	××	1900	×
Sauce, Asia at home, chilli, ¼ cup	0	0		190	
Sauce, barbecue, 1 tbsp	0	0		145	×
Sauce, Bearnaise, 2 tbsp	0	18.0	××	715	
Sauce, Bechamel, 2 tbsp	0	10.0	××	465	
Sauce, beef & black bean, ½ cup	n/a	1.0	✓	270	

Food	Fibre g	Fat g	Fat Rating	Energy kJ	Carb Rating
Sauce, Bolognaise, average serve, 160g	2.0	17.5	×	965	
Sauce, brandy, 1/4 cup	0	19.5	××	1200	××
Sauce, butterscotch, 1/4 cup	0	16.0	××	965	××
Sauce, caramel, rich, average serve	0	35.0	××	1845	××
Sauce, carbonara, average serve, 150g	0	42.0	××	1930	×
Sauce, char sui barbecue, 1 tbsp	0	0		45	×
Sauce, cheese, made from packet, 1/2 cup	0	5.0	×	440	×
Sauce, chicken & Chinese vegetables, 1/2 cup	1.0	2.0	✓	205	
Sauce, chicken tonight, average, 125g	0	1.0	×	200	×
Sauce, curry, green Thai, 1 serve, 93g	1.0	6.0	✓	420	×
Sauce, curry, green Thai, with coconut cream, 1 serve	1.0	32.0	××	1500	×
Sauce, curry, red Thai, 1 serve, 93g	1.0	6.5	✓	525	×
Sauce, curry, red Thai, with coconut cream, 1 serve	1.0	32.5	××	1610	×
Sauce, custard, ½ cup	0	5.0	×	435	✓
Sauce, hard, 2 tbsp	0	10.0	××	960	××
Sauce, honey mustard, ½ cup	0	14.0	××	750	×
Sauce, kecap manis, 1 tbsp	0	0		365	×
Sauce, korma curry, packet, made up, ½ cup	1.0	18.0	✓	920	×
Sauce, lemon chicken with vegetables, 1/2 cup	1.0	0		365	×
Sauce, marinara (for pasta), no cream, average serve	1.0	3.0	✓	645	✓
Sauce, mint, 2 teaspoons	0	0		40	
Sauce, Mongolian lamb, 1/2 cup	0	0.5		430	×
Sauce, Moroccan, Neil Perry, 50g	0	2.5	✓	145	
Sauce, mushroom, average serve for pasta	8.0	7.0	✓	1750	
Sauce, mustard, 1 tbsp	0	0		110	×
Sauce, onion, made from powder, 1/2 cup	0	1.0	×	145	×
Sauce, parsley, made from powder, 1/2 cup	0	5.0	×	505	×
Sauce, peanut, 1/4 cup	3.5	24.0	×	1100	
Sauce, pesto, 1/4 cup	1.0	45.0	✓✓	1740	

Food	Fibre g	Fat g	Fat Rating	Energy kJ	Carb Rating
Sauce, rich 4 cheese, for pasta, 150g	0	33.0	×	1630	
Sauce, rich Neapolitan (for pasta), 1 cup	3.5	10.0	×	540	
Sauce, rich Sicilian tomato (for pasta), 1 cup	3.0	13.0	✓	615	✓
Sauce, satay, home-made, 1/2 cup	4.0	29.0	×	1420	
Sauce, satay, thin, prepared, 1/2 cup	2.0	6.5	×	365	×
Sauce, soy, 1 tbsp	0	0		60	
Sauce, spicy plum with vegetables, 1/2 cup	1.0	0		420	×
Sauce, spicy red, 1 tbsp	0	0		60	
Sauce, steak, 1 tbsp	0	0		120	×
Sauce, sweet and sour plum, ½ cup	0	0.5		595	×
Sauce, sweet 'n' sour with vegetables, 1/2 cup	1.0	0		545	×
Sauce, taco bean, average serve, 160g	7.0	4.0	✓	515	✓
Sauce, tomato, 1 tbsp	0.5	0		85	
Sauce, tomato, home-made, for pasta, 1 cup	7.5	5.0	✓	520	✓
Sauce, tomato, ready-made, for pasta, 1 cup	5.5	2.0	✓	630	✓
Sauce, white, 1/4 cup	0	5.5	×	365	×
Sauce, Worcestershire, 1 tbsp	0	0		60	
Sausage roll, 1, 130g	1.5	23.0	××	1560	×
Sausage roll, party, 42g	0.5	8.5	×	530	×
Sausage roll, short pastry, 1 small, 60g	1.0	19.0	××	1150	×
Sausage, beef, grilled, 1, 80g	2.0	14.5	×	855	
Sausage, Berliner, 100g	1.0	18.0	××	945	
Sausage, black pudding, grilled, 100g	2.0	23.5	××	1310	
Sausage, chicken, 2 small, 170g	0	28.0	×	1500	
Sausage, chipolata, extra lean, 100g	0	8.0	×	620	
Sausage, Chorizo, 100g	0	38.0	×	1900	
Sausage, devon/fritz, 50g	0.5	9.0	××	490	
Sausage, frankfurt, cooked, 1, 105g	2.0	21.0	××	1090	
Sausage, garlic (sandwich), 50g	1.0	9.5	×	515	
Sausage, ham & chicken luncheon, 50g	1.0	9.0	×	480	
Sausage, Kabana, 50g	0	12.5	××	585	

Food	Fibre g	Fat g	Fat Rating	Energy kJ	Carb Rating
Sausage, Mortadella, 50g	0.5	14.5	××	675	
Sausage, Nutri-lean, 100g	0	3.0	×	450	
Sausage, polony, 50g	0	10.5	××	585	
Sausage, pork, extra lean, 100g	0	8.0	×	665	
Sausage, pork, grilled, 1, 80g	1.0	17.5	×	950	
Sausage, saveloy, battered, 1, 120g	0.5	25.0	××	1535	×
Sausage, spam, canned, 50g	0	15.5	××	690	
Sausage, Strasbourg, 50g	1.0	9.5	×	510	
Sausage, white, 100g	3.0	36.0	×	1875	
Sausages, vegetarian, 2 small, 75g	1.5	10.0	✓	635	✓
Saveloy, battered, 1, 120g	0.5	25.0	××	1535	
Savoury Indian snack mix, 25g	1.5	8.0	×	525	×
Savoury rice, 1 cup	2.0	6.0	×	800	✓
Scallops in garlic butter sauce	0	21.0	×	1030	
Scallops, Tasmanian, 6	0	0.5	✓	200	
Scampi, crumbed, fried, 2, 100g	1.0	17.5	×	1320	
Schnitzel, veal, frozen, fried, 145g	1.5	39.0	×	2030	
Schnitzel, veal, home-made, average piece, 190g	0.5	27.0	×	1660	×
Schnitzel, vegetarian, frozen, 1, 100g	2.0	16.0	✓	1100	✓
Scone, cheese, purchased, 1, 85g	1.5	10.0	×	1180	✓
Scone, date, purchased, 1, 85g	3.0	4.5	×	1080	✓
Scone, fruit, purchased, 1, 85g	2.5	4.5	×	1140	✓
Scone, home-made, 1, 45g	1.0	4.0	×	530	✓
Scone, home-made, wholemeal, 1, 50g	2.5	7.0	×	685	✓
Scotch egg, 1	0.5	39.0	×	2070	×
Scrambled egg McMuffin, 1 serve, 160g	3.5	16.5	×	1405	✓
Scrambled eggs, 2	0	18.0	×	860	
Seafood sticks, 100g	0	0.5		290	
Seasoning, stir-fry Szechwuan, 1 tbsp	0	0.5		215	×
Seasoning, stir-fry wet mix, 1 tbsp	0.5	0.5		205	×
Seaweed agar, raw, 2 tbsp, 10g	0	0		10	

Food	Fibre g	Fat g	Fat Rating	Energy kJ	Carb Rating
Seaweed, agar, dried, 10g	1.0	0		130	
Seaweed, Irish moss, raw, 2 tbsp, 10g	0	0		20	
Seaweed, kelp, raw, 10g	0	0		20	
Seaweed, kombu, dried, raw, 10g	6.0	0		20	
Seaweed, laver, raw, 10 sheets	0.5	0		40	
Seaweed, nori, dried, 10 sheets, 5g	2.5	0		30	
Seaweed, spirulina, dried, ¼ cup, 4g	0	0.5		50	
Seaweed, spirulina, raw, 10g	0	0		10	
Seaweed, wakame, dried, raw, 10g	4.5	0.5		30	
Semolina gnocchi with Parmesan, 300g	0.5	29.0	✗	1590	✓
Semolina, 100g dry	3.0	1.0	✓	1350	✓
Semolina, cooked, 1 cup, 230g	1.5	0		295	✓
Sesame oil, 1 tbsp	0	20.0	✓	740	
Sesame paste, 1 tbsp 20g	1.0	10.0	✓	600	
Sesame seed health bar, 45g	3.5	12.0	✓	700	✗
Sesame seeds, 1 tbsp 10g	1.0	5.5	✓	245	
Sesame tahini paste, 1 tbsp, 20g	1.0	9.5	✓	480	
Seven-Up soft drink, 1 can, 370 mL	0	0		650	✗✗
Shallots, 4, 25g	0.5	0		25	
Shapes with spring onion dip, 1, 55g	1.0	12.5	✗✗	820	✗
Shark, angel, (flake), grilled, 150g	0	0.5	✓	620	
Shepherd's pie, home-made, average serve, 280g	2.0	24.0	✗✗	1680	✓
Shepherd's pie, take-away, average serve, 275g	2.0	17.0	✗✗	1390	✓
Sherry, dry, 1 glass, 60 mL	0	0		285	
Sherry, medium dry, 1 glass, 60 mL	0	0		290	
Sherry, sweet, 1 glass, 60 mL	0	0		335	
Shortbread biscuits, commercial, 2, 35g	0.5	8.5	✗✗	720	✗✗
Shortbread, home-made, 30g piece	0.5	6.5	✗✗	550	✗✗
Shortcrust pastry, frozen, raw, 75g	1.5	21.5	✗✗	1375	✗
Shortcrust pastry, home-made, 1/8 20cm pie	2.0	19.0	✗✗	1450	✗

Food	Fibre g	Fat g	Fat Rating	Energy kJ	Carb Rating
Shredded wheat, 2 biscuits, 50g	6.5	0.5		665	✓
Sicilian tomato sauce, (for pasta), 1 cup	3.0	13.0	✓	615	✓
Silver bream, 150g	0	4.5	✓✓	660	
Silverbeet, cooked, 1/2 cup, 60g	2.0	0		45	
Silverside, corned, boiled, lean & fat, 2 slices, 85g	0	11.0	✗	725	
Silverside, corned, boiled, lean only, 2 slices, 80g	0	3.0	✗	435	
Singapore Sling, 150 mL	0	0		935	✗
Sirloin steak, grilled, lean & fat, 1 steak, 135g	0	26.0	✗	1550	
Sirloin steak, grilled, lean only, 1 steak, 110g	0	10.0	✗	890	
Skirt steak, raw, lean & fat, 100g	0	3.5	✗	515	
Skirt steak, raw, lean only, 100g	0	2.5	✗	470	
Skittles confectionery, 1, 60g	0	4.5	✗✗	1025	✗✗
Smarties, 50g packet	0	9.0	✗✗	1000	✗✗
Smoked chicken, 75g	0	7.5	✓	520	
Smoked cod, 150g	0	2.0	✓✓	595	
Smoked mussels, 100g can, drained, 65g	0	8.5	✓✓	530	
Smoked oysters, 100g can, drained, 65g	0	8.0	✓✓	565	
Smoked salmon, 50g	0	2.5	✓✓	280	
Smoked turkey, 75g	0	1.0	✓	300	
Smoothie, banana, 1 large glass	2.0	11.0	✗	1300	✓
Smoothie, soy banana & mango, 1 cup, 250 mL	0	4.0	✓	750	✓
Smoothie, strawberry, 275 mL	2.0	11.0	✗	1200	✓
Smoothie, Vaalia, 150 mL	0	0.5		420	✓
Snack and dip, smoky bacon, 1, 25g	0	5.5	✗	395	✗
Snack stop cheese 'n bacon potato mash, 1 serve	n/a	4.5	✗	935	✓
Snack stop chicken & mushroom risotto, 1 serve, 300g	n/a	5.5	✗	1170	✓
Snack stop macaroni cheese, 1 serve	n/a	8.0	✗	1430	✓
Snack stop spaghetti & meatballs, 1 serve, 300g	n/a	12.0	✗	1380	✓

Food	Fibre g	Fat g	Fat Rating	Energy kJ	Carb Rating
Snake beans, 100g	3.0	0		95	
Snapper, grilled, 150g	0	1.0	✓✓	590	
Snickers bar, 1, 60g	1.5	13.5	✗✗	1190	✗✗
Snow peas, 50g	2.0	0		80	
So Good drinks, see under soy					
So Good mango ice cream, 100g	0	2.0	✓	460	✗
Soba noodle salad, entree size	4.0	42.0	✓	1940	✓✓
Soba or udon buckwheat noodles, 100g dry	1.5	2.0	✓	1520	✓✓
Soda bread, 1/10 25cm loaf	4.5	7.0	✗	1275	✓
Soda water, 1 glass	0	0		0	
Soft drink, cola, 1 can, 370 mL	0	0		650	✗✗
Soft drink, diet, average, 1 can, 370 mL	0	0		15	
Soft drink, dry ginger ale, 1 glass, 250 mL	0	0		295	✗✗
Soft drink, lemon flavour, 1 can, 370 mL	0	0		735	✗✗
Soft drink, lemonade, 1 glass, 250 mL	0	0		440	✗✗
Soft drink, Lucozade, 250 mL	0	0		720	✗✗
Soft drink, mineral water & juice, 1 can, 370 mL	0	0		590	✗✗
Soft drink, orange flavour, 1 can, 370 mL	0	0		820	✗✗
Soft drink, sarsparilla, 1 can, 370 mL	0	0		730	✗✗
Soft drink, Seven-Up, 1 can, 370 mL	0	0		650	✗✗
Soft drink, tonic water, 1 glass, 250 mL	0	0		375	✗✗
Soft serve, see frozen yoghurt and ice cream					
Soft serve, Vitari, 1 cone	0	0		275	✗✗
Sorbet, commercial, 100g	0	0		560	✗✗
Sorbet, lemon, average serve, 100g	0	1.5	✗	485	✗✗
Souffle, cheese, average serve	0.5	22.0	✗✗	1255	✗
Souffle, chocolate, restaurant, average serve	1.0	24.0	✗✗	1925	✗✗
Souffle, Grand Marnier, average serve	0.5	17.0	✗✗	1550	✗✗
Soup mix fresh vegetables, 200g	4.0	0.5		225	✓
Soup, 99% fat-free, average, 250 mL	1.5	1.0	✗	410	✓
Soup, barley & vegetable, home-made, 1 bowl	9.0	4.0	✓	995	✓✓

Food	Fibre g	Fat g	Fat Rating	Energy kJ	Carb Rating
Soup, beef consomme, 1 cup, 250 mL	0	0		135	
Soup, beef, made from packet, 1 cup	2.0	1.5	✘	190	
Soup, bouillabaisse, 1 large bowl	2.0	12.0	✓✓	1500	
Soup, canned chicken, made up, 1 cup	0	7.0	✘	550	✘
Soup, canned, cream of seafood, made up, 1 cup	1.5	7.0	✘	575	✘
Soup, canned, cream of vegetable, made up, 1 cup	1.5	6.5	✘	560	✘
Soup, chicken gumbo, 250g	1.5	1.0	✓	600	✓
Soup, chicken noodle, from packet, 1 cup	0	0.5		195	✘
Soup, chicken noodle, instant, 1 serve, 200 mL	1.5	1.0	✘	170	✘
Soup, cream of pumpkin, 250g	2.5	9.0	✘	735	✘
Soup, cream of tomato, home-made, large bowl	2.5	15.0	✘	705	✘
Soup, cream of vegetable, made from packet, 1 cup	1.5	4.0	✘	420	✓
Soup, fish chowder, average bowl	3.0	10.0	✓	850	✘
Soup, French onion, home-made, 1 bowl, 350g	1.5	7.5	✘	445	✘
Soup, French onion, made from packet, 1 cup	1.0	0		70	
Soup, gazpacho, large bowl	3.5	10.0	✓	930	✓
Soup, leek and potato, average bowl, 250g	1.5	6.0	✘	450	✓
Soup, main meal canned, 1 cup	6.5	11.5	✘	870	✓
Soup, minestrone, large bowl	5.5	7.5	✓	665	✓✓
Soup, pea & ham, canned, made up, 1 cup	5.5	2.0	✘	460	✓
Soup, pea & ham, home-made, average bowl, 450g	8.5	4.0	✘	1200	✓✓
Soup, potato & leek soup, average bowl, 250g	1.5	8.5	✘	555	✓
Soup, pumpkin, home-made,1 bowl	2.0	10.0	✘	690	✓
Soup, Thai chicken coconut, 1 bowl	0.5	42.0	✘✘	1750	✘
Soup, Thai prawn sour, 1 bowl	5.0	3.0	✓	450	
Soup, tomato, canned, made up, 1 cup	1.0	2.5	✘	450	✘
Soup, tomato, fresh, home-made, large bowl	3.0	2.5	✓	275	✓
Soup, vegetable, canned, made up, 1 cup	1.5	6.5	✘	560	✓

Food	Fibre g	Fat g	Fat Rating	Energy kJ	Carb Rating
Soup, vegetable, home-made, 350 g	9.0	1.0	✓	430	✓
Soup, vichyssoise, large bowl, 350g	2.0	18.0	××	1000	✓
Sour cream & chive snacks, 50g	1.5	8.5	×	555	×
Sour cream dip, 1 tbsp	0	3.5	××	165	
Sour cream, 1 tbsp	0	7.5	××	150	
Sour cream, 1/2 cup. 125g	0	46.0	××	1850	
Sour cream, extra lite, 1 tbsp	0	2.5	××	135	
Sour cream, lite, 1 tbsp	0	4.0	××	185	
Sour dough roll, 1, 80g	1.5	1.0	×	830	✓✓
Sour dough rye bread,, 1 slice, 60g	3.0	1.0	✓	670	✓✓
Sour dough white bread,, 1 slice, 60g	2.0	1.0	✓	640	✓✓
Sour fish soup, Vietnamese, average bowl	3.5	3.0	✓	820	
Soursop (prickly custard apple), 100g	3.5	0.5		280	✓
Souvlakia, skewered lamb, each, 60g	0	7.0	×	500	
Soy & linseed wheat bran, ¾ cup, 45g	13.5	0.5		705	✓✓
Soy bean sprouts, 1/2 cup, 30g	1.0	0		130	
Soy beans, canned in tomato sauce, 1 cup, 200g	8.5	6.0	✓✓	720	✓✓
Soy beans, canned, 1 cup, 200g	8.5	2.0	✓✓	790	✓✓
Soy beans, cooked, 1 cup, 200g	14.5	14.5	✓✓	1080	✓✓
Soy beans, dry, 1/2 cup, 100g	20.0	20.0	✓✓	1420	✓✓
Soy beans, green, 1/2 cup, 80g	3.5	5.5	✓✓	490	✓✓
Soy beans, roasted, salted, 50g	9.0	13.0	✓	985	✓
Soy burger patties, 1, 250g	15.0	12.0	✓	1130	✓
Soy cheese, 50g	0	13.5	✓	650	
Soy crisps, 50g	2.5	12.0	✓	1040	×
Soy drink, fortified, 1 cup, 250 mL	0	8.0	✓	650	✓
Soy drink, fortified, flavoured, 1 cup, 250 mL	0	8.0	✓	800	✓
Soy drink, lite, 1 cup, 250 mL	0	2.5	✓	460	✓
Soy drink, low fat, fortified, 1 cup, 250 mL	0	1.5	✓	450	✓
Soy drink, powdered, made up, 250 mL	0	4.5	✓	465	✓
Soy drink, So Good Fat free, 250 mL	0	0		400	✓

Food	Fibre g	Fat g	Fat Rating	Energy kJ	Carb Rating
Soy drink, So Good Lite, 250 mL	0	1.5	✓	450	✓
Soy drink, So Good Smoothie, 250 mL	0	4.0	✓	750	✓
Soy drink, So Good, 250 mL	0	8.5	✓	650	✓
Soy drink, So Natural, 250 mL	12.0	18.0	✓	1665	✓
Soy drink, Soy Life, 1 cup, 250 mL	0	8.5	✓	715	✓
Soy drink, Soy Life, low-fat, 1 cup, 250 mL	0	2.5	✓	475	✓
Soy drink, unfortified, 1 cup, 250 mL	0	5.5	✓	410	✓
Soy sauce, 1 tbsp	0	0		30	
Soy yoghurt, fruit flavoured, 200g	8.0	5.0	✓	720	×
Soy yoghurt, vanilla, 200g	8.0	4.5	✓	760	×
Soy, Good Life, 1 cup, 250 mL	0	2.5	✓	450	✓
Soybean oil, 1 tbsp	0	20.0	✓	740	
Space food sticks, 1, 17g	0	3.0	×	300	××
Spaghetti - see also pasta					
Spaghetti & meat sauce, canned, 1/2 can, 220g	2.0	5.0	×	655	✓
Spaghetti Bolognaise, average serve	5.0	33.0	×	2800	✓
Spaghetti marinara (no cream), average serve	6.0	9.0	✓	2110	✓✓
Spaghetti squash, cooked, 1 cup, 150g	3.0	0.5		145	
Spaghetti, canned, tomato sauce, 1/2 can, 220g	2.0	1.0	✓	560	×
Spaghetti, cooked, 1 cup, 140g	2.5	0.5		695	✓✓
Spaghetti, dry, 100g	5.0	2.0	✓	1455	✓✓
Spaghetti, wholemeal, cooked, 1 cup, 150g	6.0	1.5	✓	725	✓✓
Spaghetti, wholemeal, dry, 100g	11.5	2.5	✓	1380	✓✓
Spam sausage, canned, 50g	0	15.5	××	690	
Spanakopita, frozen, 1, 120g	1.5	24.5	×	1465	×
Special K, 1 cup, 40g	1.0	0		630	✓
Spinach & cheese filled pasta, as purchased, 125g	2.0	7.0	×	1625	×
Spinach pie (spanakopita), 1/6 pie	6.0	42.0	×	2150	×
Spinach pie, Lebanese, 1 slice, 100g	3.0	20.5	×	1215	×
Spinach, cooked, 1/2 cup, 70g	4.5	0		55	

Food	Fibre g	Fat g	Fat Rating	Energy kJ	Carb Rating
Spinach, frozen, cooked, 1/2 cup, 95g	4.5	0.5		85	
Spinach, raw, 1 cup, 35g	1.0	0		20	
Spinach, water, raw, 1 cup, 35g	1.0	0		30	
Spirits, brandy, 1 0nip, 30 mL	0	0		255	
Spirits, gin, 1 nip, 30 mL	0	0		270	
Spirits, rum, 1 nip, 30 mL	0	0		265	
Spirits, vodka, 1 nip, 30 mL	0	0		265	
Spirits, whisky, 1 nip, 30 mL	0	0		270	
Spirulina, dried, ¼ cup, 4g	0	0.5		50	
Spirulina, dried, 10g	0.5	0.5		120	
Spirulina, raw, 10g	0	0		10	
Splenda sweetener, 1 teaspoon	0	0		10	
Split peas, green & yellow, cooked, 1 cup, 170g	6.5	0.5		410	✓✓
Split peas, green & yellow, dry, 100g	10.0	2.0	✓	1240	✓✓
Sponge fingers, 2, 24g	0	1.5	×	350	××
Sponge pudding, canned, 75g	2.0	8.5	××	900	××
Sponge, Genoise, 1/10 cake	0.5	7.0	××	680	××
Sponge, jam filled, 1 slice, 45g	0.5	2.0	××	575	××
Sponge, plain, purchased, 1/8 cake, 50g	0.5	2.0	××	625	××
Sponge, vanilla, purchased, 1/8 cake, 50g	0.5	7.0	××	675	××
Sponge, Victoria, 1/10 cake	1.0	23.0	××	1670	××
Spreads, see margarine, butter					
Spring greens, cooked, 1 cup, 110g	6.5	0.5		90	
Spring onions, 4, 50g	1.0	0		55	
Spring roll wrappers, 18cm square, 1, 32g	0.5	0.5		390	×
Spring roll, commercial, 1, 160g	2.0	16.0	××	1525	×
Spring rolls, home-made, each	3.0	33.0	××	1900	×
Spring rolls, mini, 50g	0.5	5.0	×	475	×
Squash, acorn, average serve, 65g	2.0	0		150	
Squash, button, cooked, 2, 70g	2.0	0		80	
Squash, scallopini, cooked, 1 medium, 80g	1.5	0		70	

Food	Fibre g	Fat g	Fat Rating	Energy kJ	Carb Rating
Squash, spaghetti, cooked, 1 cup, 150g	3.0	0.5		145	
Squid rings, battered and fried, 150g	1.0	23.5	×	1225	×
Squid rings, frozen, 100g	0	1.0	✓✓	280	
Squid, fresh, 100g	0	1.0	✓✓	330	
Squid, stuffed, average serve	2.5	8.5	✓✓	750	✓
Steak and kidney pie, average serve	1.5	50.0	×	3520	×
Steak and kidney pudding, 1/6 pie	2.0	39.0	×	2830	×
Steak Diane, medium fillet	0	29.0	×	1650	
Stock cube, 1, 5g	0	0.5		45	
Stock, chicken, ready made, 1 cup	0	0.5		95	
Stock, concentrated, 1 sachet, average	0	0		30	
Stock, vegetable, ready made, 1 cup	0	2.0	✓	160	
Stout (5.7% alc.), 1 middie, 280 mL	0	0		640	
Stout (5.7% alc.), 1 middie, 280 mL	0	0		640	
Strasbourg sausage, 50g	1.0	9.5	×	510	
Strawberries, 1/2 punnet, 125g	3.0	0		100	✓
Strawberries, canned, syrup drained, 1 cup, 250g	9.0	0		815	✓
Strawberries, frozen, 100g	4.0	0		145	✓
Strawberry jam, home-made, 1 tbsp	0	0		170	×
Strawberry shake, regular	0	15.5	×	2070	✓
Strawberry shortcake, average serve	3.0	28.0	××	2000	××
Stroganoff, beef, average serve, 1 1/2 cups	2.5	48.0	×	2620	
Stuffed tomatoes, large, each	3.5	2.0	✓	570	✓
Stuffed vine leaves, 3 average	2.0	15.0	✓	790	✓
Stuffed zucchini, each, 200g	2.5	11.0	××	1070	✓
Stuffing mix, 50g dry	4.0	0.5		680	×
Stuffing, average, 60g serve	1.5	5.0	×	470	×
Subway, 7 under 6, Ham Deli, 1	n/a	3.5	✓	910	✓
Subway, 7 under 6, Ham, 1	n/a	4.5	✓	1180	✓
Subway, 7 under 6, Roast beef Deli, 1	n/a	3.5	✓	910	✓

Food	Fibre g	Fat g	Fat Rating	Energy kJ	Carb Rating
Subway, 7 under 6, Roast beef, 1	n/a	4.5	✓	1180	✓
Subway, 7 under 6, Roasted chicken, 1	n/a	5.5	✓	1350	✓
Subway, 7 under 6, Subway Club, 1	n/a	5.5	×	1240	✓
Subway, 7 under 6, Turkey breast & ham, 1	n/a	5.0	✓	1190	✓
Subway, 7 under 6, Turkey breast deli, 1	n/a	4.0	×	930	✓
Subway, 7 under 6, Turkey breast, 1	n/a	6.0	✓	1210	✓
Subway, 7 under 6, Veggie Delite, 1	n/a	3.5	✓	990	✓
Subway, bread, deli style roll, 1	n/a	2.5	×	740	✓
Subway, bread, Hearty Italian, 15cm roll	n/a	4.0	×	1390	✓
Subway, bread, Honey Oat, 15cm roll	n/a	3.5	×	1010	✓
Subway, bread, Parmesan Oregano, 15cm roll	n/a	4.5	×	960	✓
Subway, bread, Wheat, 15cm roll	n/a	3.0	✓	870	✓
Subway, bread, White, 15cm roll	n/a	3.0	✓	900	✓
Subway, classic, Chicken fillet, 1	n/a	20.0	×	1860	✓
Subway, classic, Italian BMT, 1	n/a	25.0	×	2040	✓
Subway, classic, Meatball, 1	n/a	23.0	×	1970	✓
Subway, classic, Seafood & Crab, 1	n/a	14.0	✓	1680	✓
Subway, classic, Subway Melt, 1	n/a	18.0	×	1760	✓
Subway, classic, Tuna Deli, 1	n/a	12.0	✓	1320	✓
Subway, classic, Tuna, 1	n/a	15.0	✓	1730	✓
Subway, cookie, chewy chocolate chip,1	n/a	7.0	×	690	✓
Subway, cookie, double chocolate chip,1	n/a	8.0	×	700	✓
Subway, Salads, classic, Italian BMT, 1	n/a	19.0	×	1140	✓
Subway, Salads, classic, Steak & Cheese, 1	n/a	8.0	×	690	✓
Subway, Salads, classic, Subway Melt, 1	n/a	12.0	×	850	✓
Subway, Salads, classic, Subway Melt, 1	n/a	12.0	×	850	✓
Subway, Salads, classic, Tuna, 1	n/a	9.0	✓	820	✓
Subway, Salads, low fat, Roast Chicken, 1	n/a	2.5	✓	580	✓
Subway, Salads, low fat, Subway Club, 1	n/a	3.0	✓	470	✓
Subway, Salads, low fat, Turkey breast & Ham, 1	n/a	2.5	✓	410	✓
Subway, Salads, low fat, Veggie Delite, 1	n/a	1.0	✓	210	✓

Food	Fibre g	Fat g	Fat Rating	Energy kJ	Carb Rating
Subway, Sauces, Dijon Horseradish, 23mL	n/a	10.0	✓	390	✓
Subway, Sauces, Honey Mustard, 23mL	n/a	0.5		150	✓
Subway, Select 15cm, Caesar Chicken, 1	n/a	15.0	✓	1670	✓
Subway, Select 15cm, Caesar Italian BMT, 1	n/a	18.0	×	1740	✓
Subway, Select 15cm, Chicken Satay, 1	n/a	10.0	✓	1500	✓
Subway, Select 15cm, Chicken Teriyaki, 1	n/a	5.5	×	1340	✓
Subway, Select 15cm, Dijon Horseradish Melt, 1	n/a	24.0	×	2000	✓
Subway, Select 15cm, Honey Mustard Ham, 1	n/a	5.0	✓	1330	✓
Subway, Select 15cm, Southwest steak & cheese, 1	n/a	19.0	×	1840	✓
Suet mix, 100g	0	53.0	××	2660	
Sugar snap peas, 100g	4.0	0		145	
Sugar, any type, 1 level tsp, 5g	0	0		80	××
Sugar, any type, 1 tbsp, 20g	0	0		400	××
Sukiyaki, average serve	3.5	21.0	✓	1870	
Sultana Bran, 1 cup, 45g	6.5	1.0	✓	640	✓✓
Sultanas, 30g	1.5	0		385	✓
Summer pudding with cream	9.5	26.0	××	1995	✓
Summer pudding, average serve	9.5	1.5	✓	1075	✓
Sundae, ice cream with hot fudge, average	1.0	59.0	××	3000	××
Sun-dried tomato paste, 2 tsp	0.5	4.5	✓	220	✓
Sun-dried tomato pesto, 2 tsp	0.5	7.5	✓	385	
Sun-dried tomato, 3 pieces, 6g	1.0	0		65	
Sun-dried tomatoes in canola oil, 50g	3.0	11.0	✓	660	✓
Sun-dried tomatoes in oil, drained, 50g	3.0	7.0	✓	445	✓
Sunflower & honey health bar, 1, 50g	4.0	9.5	✓	650	×
Sunflower oil, 1 tbsp	0	20.0	✓✓	740	
Sunflower seeds, 1 tbsp, 15g	1.5	7.0	✓✓	345	
Surimi fish stick, crab-flavoured, 3, 105g	0	1.0	✓	400	
Sushi, 4 pieces	1.0	1.0	✓	575	✓
Sustagen Gold, 250 mL	0	9.0	×	1170	×

Food	Fibre g	Fat g	Fat Rating	Energy kJ	Carb Rating
Sustagen light, any flavour, 250 mL	0	2.0	×	340	×
Sustain, 1 cup, 60g	4.5	1.5	✓	940	✓
Swede, cooked, 1/2 cup, 75g	2.0	0		65	✓
Sweet & sour pork, average serve	0.5	52.0	×	2700	×
Sweet & sour sauce, take-away 1/2 cup	0	4.0	×	830	×
Sweet potato, baked, average piece, 100g	2.0	8.0	×	600	✓
Sweet potato, orange, cooked, average piece, 100g	2.5	0		275	✓✓
Sweet potato, white, cooked, average piece, 100g	2.0	0		320	✓
Sweetbreads, lamb, crumbed & fried, 100g	0	14.5	×	960	
Sweetbreads, lamb, raw, 100g	0	8.0	×	550	
Sweetcorn kernels, canned, 1 cup, 125g	4.0	1.5	✓	495	✓✓
Sweetcorn, baby, canned, 6, 100g	3.5	0		75	✓
Sweetcorn, cob, 1 average, 150g without husk	5.0	1.5	✓	440	✓✓
Sweetcorn, creamed, canned, 1/2 cup, 125g	4.5	1.0	✓	425	✓
Sweetcorn, frozen cob, 1 small, 85g	4.0	1.5	✓	470	✓✓
Sweets, boiled, 4, 15g	0	0		195	××
Sweets, caramel yumbats, each, 18g	0	4.5	×	360	××
Sweets, caramels, 4, 25g	0.5	3.0	×	420	××
Sweets, chocolate creme eggs, each, 18g	0	3.0	×	290	××
Sweets, chocolate with fruit/nuts, 6 squares, 30g	1.5	9.0	×	640	××
Sweets, chocolate, dark, 6 squares, 30g	0	8.5	×	650	××
Sweets, chocolate, Lite, 75g bar	0	21.0	××	1250	××
Sweets, chocolate, milk, 10 squares, 50g	0.5	13.5	××	1080	××
Sweets, chocolate, yumbats, each square, 22.5g	0	6.0	×	485	××
Sweets, chocolates with cream filling, 2, 18g	0	4.5	×	360	××
Sweets, chocolates with cream filling, 2, 18g	0	4.5	×	360	××
Sweets, Dove milk bar, 48g	n/a	14.5	××	1060	××
Sweets, fruit gums, 6, 25g	0	0		185	××
Sweets, hard (eg Minties), 3, 14g	0	0		220	××
Sweets, jellies, 6, 30g	0	0		340	××

Food	Fibre g	Fat g	Fat Rating	Energy kJ	Carb Rating
Sweets, Kit Kat bar, 1 45g	0	12.0	××	940	××
Sweets, liquorice allsorts, 3, 24g	0	0.5		170	××
Sweets, Lite chocolate, 75g bar	0	21.0	××	1250	××
Sweets, Maltesers, 45g	n/a	9.5	××	890	××
Sweets, Mars almond bar, 1, 50g	n/a	12.5	××	1150	××
Sweets, Mars bar, 63g	1.0	11.0	××	1090	××
Sweets, Milky way bar, 1, 25g	n/a	4.0	×	455	××
Sweets, muesli bar, chocolate chip, 1, 32g	2.0	4.0	×	455	××
Sweets, muesli bar, chocolate coated, 1, 33g	1.5	6.5	×	580	××
Sweets, muesli bar, fruit, 1, 32g	1.0	4.5	×	495	××
Sweets, peppermint lifesavers, 1 packet, 20g	0	0		335	××
Sweets, peppermints, 4, 10g	0	0		165	××
Sweets, Smarties, 50g packet	0	9.0	×	1000	××
Sweets, Snickers bar, 1, 60g	n/a	13.5	××	1190	××
Sweets, toffees, 1, 25g	0	4.5	×	450	××
Sweets, Violet crumble bar, 1, 50g	0	8.0	×	885	××
Sweets, white chocolate, 50g	0	15.5	××	1105	××
Swiss Birchner muesli, average serve, 230g	6.0	8.0	✓	1220	✓✓
Swiss chard, 1/2 cup raw, 25g	0.5	0		20	
Swiss roll, 1 slice, 35g	0.5	2.5	×	480	××
Swordfish, grilled, 150g	0	11.5	✓✓	845	
Syrup, heavy (in canned fruit), 1/2 cup	0	0		465	××
Syrup, light (in canned fruit), 1/2 cup	0	0		275	××
Tabouli, 1/2 cup	6.0	11.5	✓	840	✓✓
Tabouli, Lebanese restaurant, average serve	12.0	25.0	✓	1340	✓✓
Tabouli, supermarket salad, 100g	6.0	11.0	✓	560	✓✓
Taco bean sauce (no meat), average serve, 160g	7.0	4.0	✓	515	✓
Taco shell, 1, 11g	0.5	3.0	✓	525	✓
Tacos, 1 filled shell, meat & bean sauce, 180g	3.5	14.0	××	970	✓
Tahini paste, 1 tbsp, 20g	1.6	9.5	✓	480	

Food	Fibre g	Fat g	Fat Rating	Energy kJ	Carb Rating
Tamari sauce, 1 tbsp	0	0		50	
Tamarillo, 1 medium, 90g	4.5	0		100	✓
Tamarind leaves, 1 tbsp chopped, 8g	n/a	0		40	
Tamarind pulp, (no seeds), 1 tbsp, 15g	1.0a	0		175	✓
Tamarind, fresh, 10 fruits, 60g as purchased	3.0	0.5		600	✓
Tandoori chicken, 1/4 chicken	0.5	14.0	×	1400	✓
Tandoori lamb, 200g	0.5	38.0	×	2210	✓
Tangelo, 1 medium, 130g	2.5	0		205	✓✓
Tangerine, 1 medium, 120g with skin	2.0	0		165	✓✓
Tapenade, 1/4 cup	1.5	17.0	✓	700	
Tapioca cream, average serve	1.5	14.0	×	1180	✓
Tapioca, cooked, 1 cup, 250g	1.5	0		300	✓
Tapioca, dry, 100g	4.5	0		1460	✓
Taramasalata, 1 tbsp	0	10.5	✓	415	
Taro leaves, steamed, 1/2 cup, 75g	3.0	0.5		60	
Taro, baked, 100g	4.5	0		555	✓
Taro, boiled 1/2 cup, 70g	2.0	0		310	✓
Tarragon, dried, 1 teaspoon, 2.5g	n/a	0		30	
Tart, jam, 1 small, 50g	0.5	7.5	××	745	××
Tartare sauce, 1 tbsp, 20g	0	14.0	✓	530	
Teacake, yeasted, 1 piece, 40g	1.5	3.0	×	500	✓
Tempeh, 100g	4.5	11.0	✓	810	✓
Tempura vegetable, average serve	1.0	22.0	✓	1300	
Tempura, mixed, average serve	1.0	22.0	✓	1360	
Tempura, seafood, 5 pieces	1.0	28.0	✓	2500	
Tequila Sunrise, 150 mL	0	0		650	
Teriyaki chicken, average serve	0	12.5	×	1330	
Thai beef curry, with coconut, average serve	1.5	44.0	×	2580	
Thai beef salad, average serve	4.0	8.5	×	975	
Thai Chiang mai noodles, 1 bowl, 400g	3.5	41.0	×	2400	✓
Thai chicken coconut soup, 1 bowl	0.5	42.0	××	1750	×

Food	Fibre g	Fat g	Fat Rating	Energy kJ	Carb Rating
Thai chicken curry, average serve	2.0	34.0	×	1860	✓
Thai chilli prawns, average serve	1.0	11.0	✓	815	
Thai coconut custard, 150g	0	20.0	××	1230	××
Thai coconut ice cream, 2 scoops	1.0	27.0	××	1220	××
Thai curry puffs (meat filling), each, 85g	0.5	31.0	××	1480	×
Thai fish curry, average serve	5.0	40.0	✓	3380	✓
Thai fish in tamarind sauce, 1/2 cup	1.0	13.0	✓	745	
Thai fishcakes, 3	0.5	15.0	✓	1100	×
Thai fried noodles, average serve	4.0	31.0	×	2400	✓
Thai fried rice, average serve	4.5	14.5	×	1420	✓
Thai green mango salad with pork, average serve	3.5	11.0	×	800	✓
Thai green/red curry beef, average serve	2.0	45.0	×	2300	
Thai green/red curry chicken, average serve	2.0	40.0	×	2100	
Thai noodles with vegetables, 1 cup	3.5	14.0	✓	1660	✓
Thai red pork curry, average serve, 1 cup	0.5	44.0	×	2220	✓
Thai satay sauce, 1/2 cup	4.0	29.0	××	1420	×
Thai satay, beef plus sauce, 4 skewers	5.0	42.0	×	2800	
Thai satay, chicken plus sauce, 4 skewers	5.0	37.0	×	2200	
Thai seasoning, Cuisine Essentials, 1 tbsp	0	0		40	
Thai vegetable curry with coconut, 1 cup	3.0	21.0	×	940	✓
Thai, fried tofu with peanuts, average serve	2.5	25.0	✓	1225	✓
Thick shake, chocolate, average, 300g	0	10.5	×	1410	✓
Thick shake, strawberry, average	0	15.5	×	2070	×
Thickshake, microfreeze, chocolate, 340 mL	0	9.0	×	1305	×
Thickshake, microfreeze, vanilla malt, 340 mL	0	9.0	×	1280	×
Thickshake, milk bar, 250 mL	0	15.0	×	1225	✓
Thickshake, vanilla, average	0	15.0	×	1820	✓
Thin Captain biscuits, 4, 22g	0.5	1.5	×	375	×
Thousand island dressing, 1 tbsp	0	4.5	✓	220	×
Thousand island dressing, reduced fat, 1 tbsp	0	2.0	✓	140	×

Food	Fibre g	Fat g	Fat Rating	Energy kJ	Carb Rating
Three bean mix, canned, 1 cup, 185g	11.5	0.5		665	✓✓
Thyme, dried, 1 teaspoon, 2.5g	0	0		30	
Tim Tams, each, 19g	0	5.5	✗✗	400	✗✗
Tiramisu, average serve	0	56.0	✗✗	3450	✗✗
Toad-in-the-hole, 1 sausage with batter	4.5	44.0	✗✗	2560	✗
Toasted muesli flakes, 1/2 cup, 40g	3.5	1.0	✓	560	✓
Toffee apples, each	3.0	0		650	✗
Toffee, 2.5 cm square	0	0		110	✗✗
Toffees, 1, 25g	0	4.5	✗	450	✗✗
Tofu ice dessert, low fat, 100g	0	4.0	✓	515	✗✗
Tofu ice dessert, soft serve, average, 110g	0	8.0	✓	660	✗✗
Tofu, dried, fu juk, 100g	2.0	16.0	✓	1620	
Tofu, fermented, salted, 100g	0.5	8.0	✓	485	
Tofu, firm, 100g	0	2.5	✓	260	
Tofu, firm, nigari, 100g	0.5	4.5	✓	320	
Tofu, fried, 100g	1.0	18.0	✓	1085	
Tofu, natural organic, 100g	0	1.5	✓	370	
Tofu, silken, 100g	0	2.5	✓	230	
Tofu, Soyco, 100g	1.5	9.5	✓	730	
Tofu, stir-fried with vegetables, average serve	0	10.0	✓	520	
Tomato cream soup, home-made, large bowl	2.5	15.0	✗✗	705	
Tomato juice, 250 mL	1.0	0		200	✓
Tomato paste, 1 tbsp	0.5	0		50	
Tomato puree, 1 cup, 250g	5.0	0		300	✓
Tomato relish, home-made, 1 tbsp	0.5	0		80	
Tomato sauce, 1 tbsp	0.5	0		85	
Tomato sauce, for pasta, ready-made, 1 cup	5.5	2.0	✓	630	✓
Tomato sauce, home-made, for pasta, 1 cup	7.5	8.0	✓	820	✓
Tomato, cherry, 6, 100g	1.5	0		50	
Tomato, egg-shaped, 1 medium, 75g	1.0	0		45	
Tomato, large, stuffed (rice/nut filling) 1	3.5	2.0	✓	570	✓

Food	Fibre g	Fat g	Fat Rating	Energy kJ	Carb Rating
Tomato, raw, 1 large, 220g	2.5	0		125	
Tomato, raw, 1 medium, 160g	2.0	0		90	
Tomato, raw, 1 small, 100g	1.0	0		55	
Tomato, soup, canned, made up, 1 cup	1.0	2.5	×	450	×
Tomato, soup, fresh, home-made, large bowl	3.0	2.5	✓	275	✓
Tomato, sun dried, in oil, drained, 3 pieces, 30g	1.0	4.5	✓	270	
Tomato, sun-dried paste, 2 tsp	0.5	4.5	✓	220	✓
Tomato, sun-dried, ½ cup, 27g	3.5	1.0	✓	290	✓
Tomato, sun-dried, 3 pieces, 6g	1.0	0		65	
Tomato, sun-dried, in oil, drained, 50g	3.0	7.0	✓	445	✓
Tomatoes, canned, 1 cup, including juice, 250g	3.0	0		195	✓
Tomatoes, sun-dried in canola oil, 50g	3.0	11.0	✓	660	✓
Tongue, canned, 60g	0	10.0	×	530	
Tongue, lamb, raw, fat & skin removed, 100g	0	14.5	×	835	
Tongue, ox, pickled, fat & skin removed, 100g	0	17.5	×	915	
Tongue, ox, raw, fat & skin removed, 100g	0	14.5	×	835	
Tonic water, 1 glass, 250 mL	0	0		375	××
Topping, chocolate, 2 tbsp	0	0		325	××
Topping, strawberry, 2 tbsp	0	0		300	××
Topside steak, raw, lean & fat, 100g	0	6.5	×	605	
Topside steak, raw, lean only, 100g	0	3.0	×	485	
Torte, sacher, average serve	1.5	40.0	××	2800	××
Tortellini, Barilla, 100g	2.0	14.0	×	1660	✓
Tortellini, cheese & spinach, as purchased, 100g	3.5	6.5	×	1190	✓
Tortellini, shelf-stable, 125g	3.5	5.0	×	1490	✓
Tortilla chips, 50g	4.0	11.0	✓	970	✓
Tortilla wraps, 1, 42g	1.0	2.0	×	565	✓
Tortilla, Burrito, 1, 40g	2.0	3.5	×	545	✓
Tortilla, Buttercup, 1, 50g	1.5	2.0	✓	580	✓
Tortilla, El Paso, 1, 25g	1.0	3.0	×	370	✓

Food	Fibre g	Fat g	Fat Rating	Energy kJ	Carb Rating
Tortilla, small, 1, 40g	1.0	0.5		445	✓
Tostado	21.0	35.0	××	3390	×
Treacle, 1 tbsp	0	0		220	××
Tree tomato (tamarillo), 1 medium, 90g	4.5	0		100	✓
Trifle, commercial, 125g	0.5	11.5	××	865	××
Trifle, home-made, average serve	1.0	23.0	××	2130	××
Tripe, beef, raw, 100g	0	2.0	×	300	
Tripe, cooked, 100g	0	4.5	×	420	
Triticale flour, 1 cup, 120g	12.0	4.5	✓	1810	✓
Trout, brown trout, whole, baked, 1	0	3.0	✓	660	
Tuna mornay, average serve, 200g	1.5	26.0	×	1640	✓
Tuna, canned, brine/water, 100g (drained 80g)	0	2.0	✓✓	415	
Tuna, canned, oil, 100g, (drained 80g)	0	7.5	✓✓	715	
Tuna, canned, sandwich type in oil, 100g	0	8.0	✓	780	
Tuna, canned, slices, ½ can, 65g	0	2.5	✓✓	385	
Tuna, canned, slices, smoked, ½ can, 40g	0	2.0	✓✓	260	
Tuna, fresh, grilled, 150g	0	1.0	✓✓	610	
Turkey ham, 100g	0	4.0	✓	430	
Turkey, breast fillets, 100g	0	0.5		440	
Turkey, breast roll, 100g	0	1.5	✓	495	
Turkey, breast roll, cooked, 100g	0	1.5	✓	495	
Turkey, buffe breast, skin removed, cooked, 80g	0	3.5	✓	415	
Turkey, buffe breast, smoked, cooked, no skin, 80g	0	1.0	✓	340	
Turkey, buffe breast, smoked, with skin, 80g	0	4.0	✓	440	
Turkey, buffe breast, with skin, basted, 100g	0	8.0	✓	610	
Turkey, deli, 100g	0	8.5	✓	610	
Turkey, hindquarter, meat & skin, 100g	0	13.0	×	905	
Turkey, Inghams roast, breast, 100g	0	4.0	✓	445	
Turkey, pastrami, Tegel, 50g	0	1.5	✓	230	
Turkey, raw, 100g	0	3.0	✓	450	

Food	Fibre g	Fat g	Fat Rating	Energy kJ	Carb Rating
Turkey, roast, dark meat, 100g	0	4.0	×	625	
Turkey, roast, lean only, 100g	0	4.0	✓	650	
Turkey, salami, Tegel, 50g	0	2.0	✓	240	
Turkey, smoked, breast, 100g	0	1.0	✓	395	
Turkish bread, average piece, 80g	2.0	2.0	✓	725	✓
Turkish bread, bake at home, 70g	1.5	3.0	✓	750	✓
Turkish delight, home-made, 2.5 cm square	0	0	✓	225	×
Turkish delight, purchased, 25g	0	0.5		365	××
Turnip tops, 100g	3.0	0		115	
Turnip, steamed, ½ cup, 125g	4.0	0		110	
Turtle egg, 100g	0	12.5	×	945	
Turtle, roasted, 100g	0	0.5		480	
Twisties, cheese flavoured, 50g packet	1.5	14.0	××	1065	×
Twisties, plain, 50g packet	1.5	13.5	××	1035	×
Twix confectionery, 1, 55g	1.0	13.5	××	1115	××
Two fruits, canned, 1/2 cup, 110g	2.0	0		265	✓
Two fruits, snack pack, 140g	2.5	0		335	✓
Tyropita (filo pastry, cheese & egg), 1 slice, 100g	1.0	26.0	××	1550	×
Tyropites (Greek cheese pastries), 1 small, 27g	0	6.0	×	310	×
Tzatziki (cucumber, garlic, yoghurt dip), 60g	1.0	6.5	×	330	✓
Udon noodles, Asia at Home, 150g	1.0	1.0	✓	870	✓✓
Udon noodles, flavoured, 100g	2.0	0.5		460	✓✓
Up and Go Liquid breakfast, 250 mL	3.5	4.0	✓	725	✓
Upside-side down cake, 1/8 of cake	0.5	10.0	××	750	××
Vanilla shake, regular, 418g	0	15.0	×	1820	✓
Vanilla slice, commercial, 1, 135g	0.5	12.0	××	1150	××
Vanilla syrup, 1 tbsp	0	0		60	×
Veal carbonara, average serve	0	40.0	×	2200	×
Veal Cordon Bleu	0	19.0	×	1660	×
Veal Parmigiana, average serve	3.0	55.0	×	3200	×

Food	Fibre g	Fat g	Fat Rating	Energy kJ	Carb Rating
Veal schnitzel, frozen, fried, 145g	1.5	39.0	×	2030	×
Veal schnitzel, home-made, average piece, 190g	0.5	27.0	×	1660	×
Veal, forequarter steak, raw, 100g	0	2.0	×	455	
Veal, kidneys in mustard cream sauce, average	0	35.0	×	1890	
Veal, leg steak, fried, 100g	0	3.5	×	670	
Veal, loin chop, baked or grilled, lean & fat, 2	0	5.0	×	730	
Veal, loin chop, baked or grilled, lean only, 2	0	3.0	×	620	
Veal, roasted, lean & fat, 2 slices 90g	0	1.5	×	535	
Veal, roasted, lean only, 2 slices 90g	0	1.0	×	510	
Veal, shank, cooked, lean & fat, 125g meat	0	8.0	×	930	
Veal, shank, cooked, lean only, 120 meat	0	3.0	×	735	
Vege crisps, 50g	1.5	10.5	××	1035	×
Vegeburger mix, 1/4 packet + egg, water, 1 burger	4.0	4.5	✓	600	✓
Vegemite, 1 teaspoon	0	0		20	
Vegetable juice, canned, 250 mL	2.0	0		150	
Vegetable juice, fresh, 250 mL	3.0	0		150	
Vegetable oil, 1 tbsp	0	20.0	✓✓	740	
Vegetable oil, polyunsaturated, 1 tbsp	0	20.0	✓✓	740	
Vegetable stock, ready made, 1 cup	0	2.0	✓	160	
Vegetables, see individual entries					
Vegetarian burger patties, frozen, 1, 75g	1.5	10.5	✓	740	✓
Vegetarian burgers, Zoglo, 1, 75g	1.5	5.0	✓✓	500	✓✓
Vegetarian 'chicken' patties, Zoglo, 1, 75g	1.5	4.5	✓✓	550	✓✓
Vegetarian chicken, 100g	4.5	4.5	✓	480	✓
Vegetarian hot dogs, 1, 100g	4.0	3.5	✓	675	✓
Vegetarian kabana, 50g	2.0	3.5	✓	460	✓
Vegetarian kebabs, Zoglo, 3, 125g	2.5	7.5	✓✓	805	✓✓
Vegetarian links, Zoglo, 3, 110g	2.0	7.5	✓	655	✓✓
Vegetarian meatballs, Zoglo, 2, 90g	2.0	5.5	✓✓	580	✓✓
Vegetarian multigrain patties, Zoglo, 1, 75g	2.0	2.0	✓	460	✓✓

Food	Fibre g	Fat g	Fat Rating	Energy kJ	Carb Rating
Vegetarian not bacon, 50g	3.0	7.5	✓	565	✓
Vegetarian not burgers, 100g	4.0	5.0	✓	815	✓
Vegetarian nuggets, Zoglo, 4, 140g	1.5	7.0	✓	590	✓✓
Vegetarian party franks, 100g	4.0	3.5	✓	675	✓
Vegetarian patties, Zoglo, 2, 150g	3.0	10.5	✓	1000	✓✓
Vegetarian sausages, frozen, 2, 75g	1.5	10.0	✓	635	✓
Vegetarian schnitzel, frozen, 1, 100g	2.0	16.0	✓	1100	✓
Vegetarian schnitzel, Zoglo, 1, 100g	2.0	10.0	✓	845	✓✓
Venison, roast, 100g	0	3.0	✓	660	
Vermicelli, dry, 100g	5.0	0.5		1485	✓
Vermouth, dry, 1 glass, 60 mL	0	0		295	
Vermouth, sweet, 1 glass, 60 mL	0	0		380	
Vichyssoise, large bowl, 350g	2.0	18.0	✗	1000	✓
Vindaloo curry sauce, with coconut milk, ¼ packet	0	25.0	✗✗	1145	✗
Vine leaves, preserved in brine, 6, 18g	1.0	0		10	
Vine leaves, stuffed, 4, 140g	1.5	4.0	✓	635	✓
Vinegar, 1 tbsp	0	0		15	
Violet crumble bar, 1, 50g	0	8.0	✗✗	885	✗✗
Vita Brits, 2 biscuits, 33g	4.0	0.5		500	✓
Vita Wheat, 4, 25g	3.0	2.5	✓	410	✓
Vitari, average serve	0	0		235	✗
Vodka, 1 nip, 30 mL	0	0		265	
Vol au vent, 1, 130g	1.0	22.5	✗✗	1335	✗
Waffles with ice cream and syrup, average serve	1.0	17.0	✗✗	1820	✗✗
Waffles, frozen, 1	0	1.0	✗	195	✗
Waffles, home-made, each	1.5	18.0	✗✗	1440	✗
Waffles, purchased, 1, 34g	0.5	5.5	✗	475	✗
Wagon wheels, 1	0.5	4.5	✗	450	✗✗
Wakame, (seaweed), dried, raw, 10g	4.5	0.5		30	
Waldorf salad, average serve, 140g	3.0	18.0	✓	995	✓

Food	Fibre g	Fat g	Fat Rating	Energy kJ	Carb Rating
Walnut oil, 1 tbsp	0	20.0	✓✓	740	
Walnuts, 1/2 cup, 50g	3.0	35.0	✓✓	1425	
Wasabi, 1g	0	0		5	
Water biscuits, 2, 15g	1.0	2.0	×	280	×
Water chestnuts, canned, ½ cup	1.5	0		125	✓
Water lily root, 100g	n/a	0		865	✓
Watercress, 1 cup leaves, 35g	1.5	0		30	
Watermelon seed kernels, dried, 1/4 cup, 25g	n/a	12.0	✓	630	✓
Watermelon, 1 cup cubed, 180g	1.0	0		155	✓
Wattle seed, 1 tbsp	9.0	2.0	✓	305	✓
Wax jambu, 1 medium, 35g	0.5	0		35	
Weeta Puffs, 1 cup, 20g	1.0	0.5		295	✓
Weetbix Hi-Bran & soy, 2 biscuits, 40g	7.0	2.5	✓	520	✓
Weetbix-Bix plus oatbran, 2 biscuits, 40g	5.5	1.5	✓	535	✓
Weetbix-Bix, 2 biscuits, 30g	3.5	0.5		420	✓
Weeties, 1 cup, 35g	4.5	1.0	✓	455	✓
Welsh rarebit, 2 slices	1.5	21.0	×	1250	✓
Wheat bran, unprocessed, 2 tbsp, 12g	5.5	0.5		80	
Wheat flakes, 1 cup, 45g	5.5	1.0	✓	600	✓
Wheat, rolled, ½ cup, 80g	7.0	1.5	✓	1140	✓✓
Wheatgerm & fruit health bar, 1, 45g	3.5	8.0	×	590	×
Wheatgerm oil, 1 tbsp	0	20.0	✓✓	740	
Wheatgerm, 2 tbsp, 18g	3.5	1.5	✓✓	200	
Whisky, 1 nip, 30 mL	0	0		270	
White chocolate, 50g	0	15.5	××	1105	××
White radish, 1 cup sliced, 100g	1.5	0.5		70	
White rice & wild rice blend, 100g	1.5	1.0	✓	1480	✓
White Russian, 90 mL	0	13.0	××	1185	
White sauce, 1/2 cup	0.5	13.5	×	735	✓
Whitebait, fried, 60g	0	28.5	✓	1305	×
Whiting, King George, grilled, 150g	0	1.0	✓✓	580	

Food	Fibre g	Fat g	Fat Rating	Energy kJ	Carb Rating
Wholemeal flour, 1 cup, 125g	17.0	3.0	✓	1755	✓
Wholemeal pastry, average portion, 65g	4.0	21.5	×	1350	✓
Wine, Champagne, 1 glass, 150 mL	0	0		405	
Wine, cooler, 1 glass, 250 mL	0	0		550	
Wine, port, 1 glass, 60 mL	0	0		375	
Wine, red, 1 glass, 150 mL	0	0		425	
Wine, rose, 1 glass, 150 mL	0	0		440	
Wine, sherry, dry, 1 glass, 60 mL	0	0		285	
Wine, sherry, medium dry, 1 glass, 60 mL	0	0		290	
Wine, sherry, sweet, 1 glass, 60 mL	0	0		335	
Wine, white, dry, 1 glass, 150 mL	0	0		415	
Wine, white, medium dry, 1 glass, 150 mL	0	0		465	
Wine, white, Sauternes, 1 glass, 150 mL	0	0		590	
Winged beans, immature seeds, cooked, ½ cup	n/a	0.5		160	
Winged beans, mature seeds, cooked, ½ cup, 85g	n/a	6.0	✓	615	✓
Winged beans, raw whole bean, 100g	n/a	0.5	✓	215	
Witchetty grub, 1, 20g	0	4.0	✓	235	
Witlof, 1 head, 60g	1.0	0		30	
Wonton wrappers, 16cm square, 1, 16g	0.5	0		200	✓
Wonton wrappers, 9cm square, 1, 8g	0	0		100	✓
Wontons, fried, each 30g	0.5	10.0	✓	485	×
Worcestershire sauce, 1 tbsp	0	0		60	
Wraps, burrito, 1, 46g	1.5	4.0	×	605	✓
Wraps, chapati, 1, 44g	2.5	4.0	✓	520	✓
Wraps, Diegos, 1, 42g	1.0	2.0	✓	565	✓
Wraps, enchilada, 1, 28g	1.0	2.5	×	365	✓
Wraps, Fajita, 1, 25g	1.0	2.5	×	340	✓
Wraps, rice paper, 1, 10g	0	0		140	✓
Wraps, roti, 1, 45g	1.5	4.0	✓	660	✓
Wraps, souvlaki, 1	2.5	5.0	×	750	✓

Food	Fibre g	Fat g	Fat Rating	Energy kJ	Carb Rating
Wraps, tortilla, 1, 42g	1.0	2.0	×	565	✓
Yabbies, 2	0	1.0	✓	320	
Yakitori, chicken, 1 skewer	0	2.0	✓	490	
Yakult, 65 mL	0	0		200	×
Yam, baked average piece, 75g	3.5	0.5		490	✓
Yam, native Australian, 100g	n/a	0		450	✓
Yam, steamed, 1/2 cup, 65g	2.5	0		320	✓
Yoghurt bars, fruitzies, apple, 1, 25g	0.5	3.5	×	440	×
Yoghurt bars, fruitzies, apricot, 1, 25g	1.0	3.5	×	390	×
Yoghurt bars, fruitzies, sultana, 1, 25g	0.5	3.5	×	450	×
Yoghurt, Activ, fibre & calcium, prune, 150g	3.0	1.5	×	655	✓
Yoghurt, Activ, strawberry, fibre & calcium, 150g	3.0	1.5	×	640	✓
Yoghurt, Activ, vanilla, 150g	0	2.5	×	890	✓
Yoghurt, Attiki, acidophilus, apricot, low-fat, 200g	0	0		465	✓
Yoghurt, Attiki, acidophilus, honey, low-fat, 200g	0	0		535	✓
Yoghurt, Attiki, acidophilus, natural, low-fat, 200g	0	0		360	✓
Yoghurt, Attiki, acidophilus, s'berry, low-fat, 200g	0	0		470	✓
Yoghurt, Bornhoffen, natural, 200g	0	7.0	×	720	✓
Yoghurt, Dairy Farmers, European, 100mL	0	8.0	×	475	✓
Yoghurt, frozen, Alfresko, 1, 180mL	0	4.0	×	595	×
Yoghurt, frozen, apricot, 85g	0	4.5	×	535	×
Yoghurt, frozen, Baskin Robbins, low-fat, 100g	0	3.0	×	480	×
Yoghurt, frozen, Baskin Robbins, non-fat, 100g	0	0		335	×
Yoghurt, frozen, fruit 'n' yoghurt, 100g	0.5	5.0	×	590	×
Yoghurt, frozen, fruit yoghurt on stick, 70g	0	2.0	×	375	×
Yoghurt, frozen, Honey Hill Farms, non-fat, 1 cone	0	1.0	×	460	×

Food	Fibre g	Fat g	Fat Rating	Energy kJ	Carb Rating
Yoghurt, frozen, Honey Hill, reduced-fat, 1 cone	0	0		380	×
Yoghurt, frozen, no fat, no sugar, 1 cone	0	0		190	✓
Yoghurt, frozen, NZ natural, 180g	0	3.5	×	1075	×
Yoghurt, frozen, Ski D'Lite, 100g	1.0	3.0	×	645	×
Yoghurt, frozen, soft serve, Colombo, 100mL	0	0.5		375	×
Yoghurt, frozen, soft serve, low-fat, average	0	3.0	×	435	×
Yoghurt, frozen, soft serve, non-fat, average	0	0		335	×
Yoghurt, fruit, 200g	0	4.0	×	740	✓
Yoghurt, fruit, low-fat, 200g	0	0.5		630	✓
Yoghurt, fruit, low-fat, no sugar, 200g	0	0.5		380	✓✓
Yoghurt, honey, European style, ½ cup	0	9.0	×	695	✓
Yoghurt, Jalna, Berry Skim, 200g	0	0		700	✓
Yoghurt, Jalna, Creamy, 200g	0	10.0	×	870	✓
Yoghurt, Jalna, Leben, 200g	0	6.5	×	660	✓
Yoghurt, Jalna, Skim, 200g	0	0		480	✓
Yoghurt, LC1, 200g	0	6.0	×	875	✓
Yoghurt, natural, 200g	0	9.0	×	715	✓✓
Yoghurt, natural, low fat, 200g	0	0.5		500	✓✓
Yoghurt, Nestle Diet, peach & mango, 200g	0	0		370	✓
Yoghurt, Nestle LC1, vanilla, 150g	0	2.0	×	655	✓
Yoghurt, Nestle Light, tropical mango, 200g	0	2.0	×	840	✓
Yoghurt, Nestle Regular, tropical mango, 200g	0	8.0	×	980	✓
Yoghurt, sheep's milk, ½ cup	0	6.0	×	440	✓
Yoghurt, Ski D'Lite, honey, 200g	0	1.5	×	870	✓
Yoghurt, soy, fruit flavoured, 200g	8.0	5.0	✓	720	×✓
Yoghurt, soy, vanilla, 200g	8.0	4.5	✓	760	×
Yoghurt, tropical fruit, low fat, 200g	0	0.5		720	×
Yoghurt, Vaalia, fruit flavours, 200g	0	3.5	×	108	✓
Yoghurt, Vaalia, natural, 200g	0	6.0	×	960	✓✓
Yoghurt, Vaalia, reduced-fat, fruit flavours, 200g	0	2.5	×	725	✓
Yoghurt, Vaalia, reduced-fat, natural, 200g	0	4.0	×	640	✓✓

Food	Fibre g	Fat g	Fat Rating	Energy kJ	Carb Rating
Yoghurt, Vaalia, reduced-fat, vanilla, 200g	0	3.0	×	845	✓
Yoghurt, Vaalia, vanilla, 200g	0	4.0	×	1265	✓
Yoghurt, vanilla, low fat, 200g	0	0.5		610	✓
Yoghurt, vanilla, natural, 200g	0	7.0	×	725	✓
Yoghurt, Vitalize Multivitamin, 200g	0	4.0	×	550	✓
Yoghurt, Y Plus, 200g	0	7.0	×	660	✓
Yoghurt, Yomix, reduced fat, fruit flavours, 200g	0	0		280	✓
Yoghurt, Yomix, reduced fat, natural, 200g	0	0		410	✓✓
Yoghurt, Yomix, reduced fat, vanilla, 200g	0	0		410	✓
Yoghurt. Greek, Peters Farm, 1/2 cup	0	6.5	×	455	✓✓
Yoghurt. Greek-style, ½ cup	0	12.0	×	750	✓✓
Yorkshire pudding, 100g	1.0	10.0	××	870	×
Yorkshire pudding, home-made, 50g	1.0	9.0	××	750	×
Zabaglione, average serve, 1/2 cup	0	8.5	×	875	×
Zoglo products, see vegetarian					
Zucchini flowers, 4	0	0		10	
Zucchini flowers, ricotta stuffing, deep fried, 4	0	16.0	✓	1020	✓
Zucchini, green, 1 medium, 90g	1.5	0		60	
Zucchini, yellow, 1 medium, 90g	1.5	0		70